ABC OF SLEEP DISORDERS

ABC OF SLEEP DISORDERS

edited by

COLIN M SHAPIRO PHD MRCPsych

Professor of psychiatry, University of Toronto, Ontario, Canada

with contributions by

WILLIAM C DEMENT, M J FLANIGAN, GERMAN E BERRIOS, COLIN A ESPIE, J D PARKES, N J DOUGLAS, T DOUGLAS BRADLEY, HELEN S DRIVER, JIM WATERHOUSE, DAVID MINORS, EILEEN P SLOAN, CAMERON G SWIFT, TONY JAFFA, STEPHEN SCOTT, JEAN HARRIS HENDRIKS, A H CRISP, P M A CALVERLEY, J R CATERALL, JAMES M KREUGER, LINDA TOTH, GERALD M DEVINS, M R G HUSSAIN, MARK KATZ, JOEL EISEN, JAMES MACFARLANE, CHRIS IDZIKOWSKI, J R STRADLING, L W REINISH, P SANDOR, PETER TYRER, R A A McCALL SMITH

Published by the BMJ Publishing Group
Tavistock Square, London WC1H 9JR

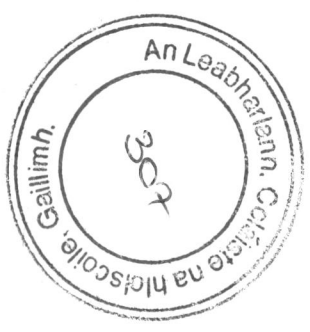

© BMJ Publishing Group 1993

First published 1993

British Library Cataloguing in Publication Data

A catalogue record for this book is available from the British Library

ISBN 0–7279–0794–8

The cover photograph was taken by Piran Murphy, with thanks to the model, Marcelle Elliot.

Printed in Great Britain by Jolly & Barber Ltd, Rugby
Typesetting by Bedford Typesetters Limited, Bedford

Contents

INTRODUCTION

Most people are fascinated by sleep. We spend a third of our lives asleep, and part of the other two thirds thinking about it. Most cultures have folk stories about sleep; painters often depict sleep, portraying the idyllic nap or the thrashing nightmare in ways that evoke the essence of the experiences. Writers have tried to plumb the mysteries of dreams only to find that they elude explanation.

Today our fascination with sleep has extended into scientific research. Sleep medicine is a new and rapidly growing specialty which is influencing the physical, psychological, and social wellbeing of an increasing number of people. Most doctors, however, have no formal training in this area and so this book has been produced specifically for them.

The *ABC of Sleep Disorders* provides a framework of perspectives of sleep, and offers a clinical approach to the most common and debilitating disruptions of sleep. I hope that it will not only supply indispensable information but also facilitate the diagnosis and proper treatment of these disorders as well as deepening understanding of patients.

The pleasure of having contributions from people who have taught me, who have been colleagues, and who until recently have been my students, is great; I pay particular tribute to Ian Oswald, who provided me with the opportunity to develop my interest in sleep and with master classes in critical evaluation.

Most of the chapters in this book have recently appeared in the *British Medical Journal*, but a number have been added, including those on aspects as diverse as the interaction between the immune system and sleep, the association between sleep and psychiatric disease, and the medicolegal aspects of sleep disorders. These chapters illustrate not only the far reaching effects of sleep disorders, but also the widening scope of this exciting new specialty.

Sleep has always been an integral part of human existence, and now more than ever is the subject of clinical and research interest. It is a great achievement to enhance a patient's sleeping hours and in doing so improve his or her waking ones as well. I thank all the authors who have contributed, and I hope that this book will contribute to the treatment of patients with sleep disorders.

I thank my former secretary, Marjorie Dodd, and my current secretary, Suzette Tumaliwan Merced, for their assistance.

COLIN M SHAPIRO

Toronto

July 1993

This book is dedicated to my children, Zoë, Gilla, and Mahla.

IMPACT AND EPIDEMIOLOGY OF SLEEP DISORDERS

Colin M Shapiro, William C Dement

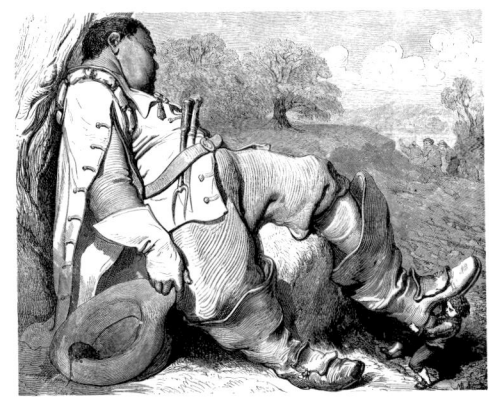

We know that one in seven Americans have a chronic sleep/wake disorder, and although similar data are not available for other Western countries the figures are probably similar. In developing countries factors such as poverty have a profound influence on sleep. In India, for example, it is estimated that one third of the population goes to sleep where they are standing when it is time to sleep.

Europe has the highest proportion of elderly people, in whom many sleep problems, such as insomnia and sleep apnoea, are more common. When taken together with the fact that hypnotics are among the most widely prescribed drugs, the impact of sleep disorders and their treatment merits particular attention in Western society. The United Kingdom, however, has lagged behind other countries in terms of developing specialised facilities for treating sleep disorders.

At present the impact of sleep disorders on morbidity and mortality is not widely appreciated. This article provides basic information about the epidemiology of a range of sleep disorders and highlights some of the implications of sleep disorders.

Impact of sleep disorders

Prevalences of some sleep disorders	
Narcolepsy	Estimated 0·15%
Obstructive sleep apnoea syndrome	4-8% of men; most common in middle aged overweight men; 2-4% of women
Restless legs syndrome	Definitive data not available; symptoms have been identified in 5-15% of normal subjects, 11% of pregnant women, 15-20% of patients with uremia, up to 30% of patients with rheumatoid arthritis
Shiftwork sleep disorder	Estimated 2-5%
Sleepwalking	1-15%; more common in children than in adults
Sleep terrors	3% of children, < 1% of adults
Nocturnal leg cramps	Definitive data not available; up to 16% of healthy people
Nightmares	10-50% of children aged 3-5 years have nightmares that disturb their parents; about 50% of adults have occasional nightmares and 1% frequent nightmares (≥ 1 a week)
Sleep paralysis	40-50% of normal subjects have isolated occurrences in lifetime; 40% of patients with narcolepsy
Impaired sleep related penile erections	> 10% men have chronic erectile dysfunction
Sleep enuresis	30% of 4 year olds, 10% of 6 year olds, 5% of 10 year olds, 3% of 12 year olds, 1-3% of 18 year olds; primary enuresis comprises 70-90% of all cases, secondary enuresis 10-30%
Insomnia	30% in one year. A third say the problem is severe
Primary snoring	40-50% of men and women > 65 years
Sudden infant death syndrome	Estimated to occur in 1-2/1000 live births
Parkinsonism (for comparison)	0·1-0·3%; may be as high as 20% of those > 60 years of age; 60-90% of people treated for Parkinson's Disease have sleep complaints

For many sleep disorders there is an associated increase in daytime sleepiness and an increase in road traffic accidents. The effect of disruption of circadian rhythms has an impact both at the time of the disruption (for example, in shift workers or the effects of jet lag) and well beyond that time—for example, there is greater sleep disruption in former shift workers 10 years after stopping shift work than in controls who have never worked shifts. It is speculative but plausible that the higher incidence of complaints of insomnia in middle aged and older women is a consequence of longstanding disrupted sleep during child rearing (at a time when the sleep drive is strong), which produces its effects 15 to 25 years later.

In many medical disorders sleep disruption makes coping with the disorder more difficult. With most sleep disorders there are many general effects—attenuation of school and work ability and opportunity, psychosocial consequences, and a constriction of leisure and pleasure time. There are specific effects linked with each condition.

Impact and epidemiology of sleep disorders

Number and cost of hypnotic drugs (BNF section) prescribed in the United Kingdom in 1989 and in Scotland alone in 1989 and 1991 (for comparison)

	No of prescriptions	Gross ingredient cost (£)
United Kingdom, 1989		
Hypnotics (4.1.1)	14 834 000	20 871 170
Anxiolytics (4.1.2)	7 586 000	6 147 590
Barbiturates (4.1.3)	306 000	516 020
Scotland, 1989 (1991)		
Hypnotics (4.1.1)	1 744 803 (1 682 256)	2 789 362 (3 255 958)
Anxiolytics (4.1.2)	850 374 (800 678)	641 607 (864 282)
Barbiturates (4.1.3)	23 985 (16 614)	39 745 (32 576)

Sleep apnoea

In the case of sleep apnoea, an association with increased risk of myocardial infarction and stroke has been reported. Cognitive deterioration, presumably on the basis of repeated nocturnal hypoxia and sleep disruption, has been described in a number of studies, and personality change, in part related to continuous fatigue, leading to marital friction and divorce or difficulties in the workplace is not uncommon. In comparison with other sleep disorders, we have recently found that this condition has more illness intrusiveness impact on the spouse than on patients with apnoea themselves.

Insomnia

There is a tendency for many doctors to trivialise the complaint of insomnia. It is an extremely common symptom and is often self-limiting. In up to 80% of cases the insomnia seen in general practice is related to anxiety and depression. Even in specialised clinics one third of insomniac patients have a psychological cause for their insomnia and if added to drugs and alcohol as causes, this would constitute half of all cases seen. Perhaps doctors' subjective experience, together with the well recognised mismatch of subjective estimates of sleep time and objective sleep time recorded by polysomnography, and the psychological emphasis in many patients has led doctors and some sleep specialists to take a minimal approach to the insomniac patient.

Only about one in 256 patients with insomnia present to their general practitioner. Of these, most raise the issue when seeing the doctor for another reason. Despite these difficulties in diagnosing and treating insomnia there are 15 million prescriptions for hypnotics in Britain annually. Many people with insomnia resort to ineffective or dangerous self-treatment regimens. The impact of sleep disruption in severe cases of insomnia can be considerable, and especially when associated with other conditions, such as Parkinson's disease, can be the trigger for suicidal behaviour.

The consequence of treatment of insomnia can be profound. Some hypnotics interact with alcohol. The impact of long term use of benzodiazepines may impair cognitive powers, especially in elderly people. However, the relief of severe insomnia both is humane and may help to prevent insomnia triggering depression or mania and a variety of illnesses.

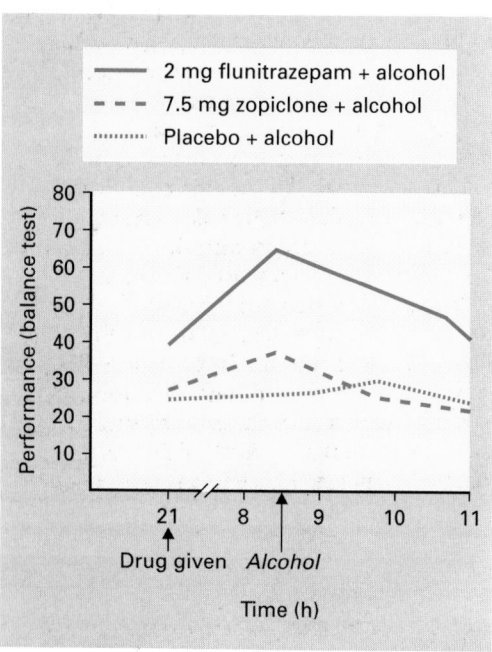

The interaction with alcohol is not the same for all hypnotics.

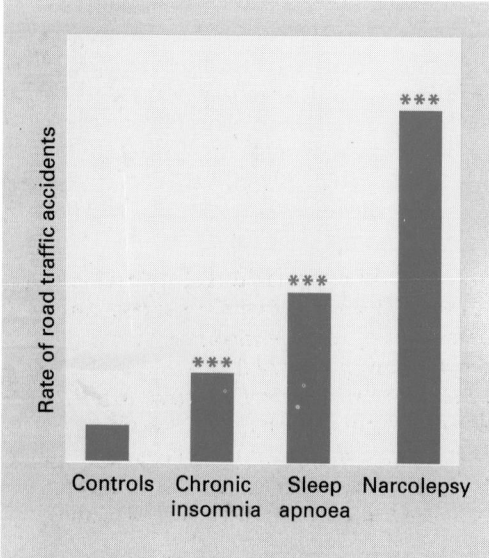

Proportional increase in the rate of road traffic accidents in patients with three sleep disorders compared with controls. (Stars indicate a high statistical significance.)

Narcolepsy

Narcolepsy is reputed to be the disorder with the longest duration from onset of symptoms to diagnosis. The treatment, with psychostimulants, carries with it specific problems. Studies of impact on quality of life for a variety of disorders, including multiple sclerosis and chronic renal failure, rate narcolepsy second only to quadraplegia.

Sleep and death

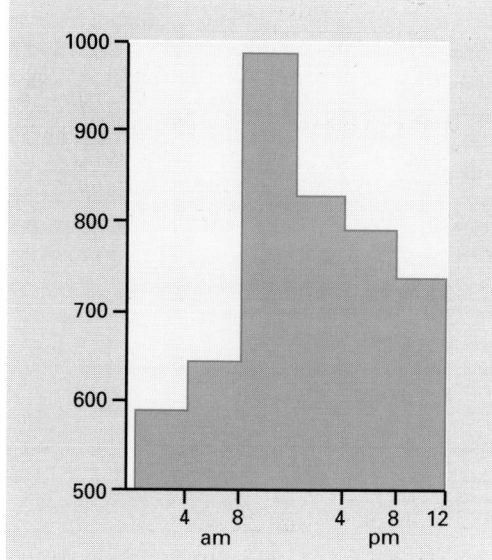

Circadian distribution of deaths from ischaemic heart disease in Scotland, 1982.

Historically, humans have held an ambivalent attitude to sleep. In Greek mythology, Nyx (Night) had two sons, Thanatos (Death) and Hypnos (Sleep). The juxtaposition of these two has led to the misconception that sleep is a passive period contrary to the recognised active restorative processes that occur in sleep.

Some authors have identified the small hours of the morning as a time of particular risk. For example, F Scott Fitzgerald wrote in 1945 "In the real dark night of the soul it is always three o'clock in the morning." Many studies show an increased mortality in the late sleep and early waking hours. Most doctors are now aware that noctural asthma is particularly pronounced in the latter part of sleep and many recognise that most REM sleep occurs in the later part of the night. These observations may be linked. Asthma, for example, is not commonly fatal, but of those dying of asthma, most die during the night. The lack of autonomic nervous system control during rapid eye movement (REM) sleep may represent a risk period for health and may be a precipitating factor in nocturnal death. Sudden infant death syndrome predominantly occurs at night and is thought to be related to pathophysiological mechanisms of sleep. There are a number of general medical disorders with peak mortality at night, as well as specific (rare) disorders associated with sleep (familial fatal insomnia, nocturnal death—especially in Southeast Asian men [Pok-kuri]—which is thought to be a REM related arrhythmia).

An American Cancer Society study of over a million volunteers followed prospectively for six years showed a 50% higher mortality in those taking sleeping pills "often" (after controlling for sleep duration). Deviation from age appropriate sleep duration leads to an increase in mortality which is more pronounced in women (168%) than in men (129%) if sleep is more than two hours shorter or longer than the norm. This effect increases with age.

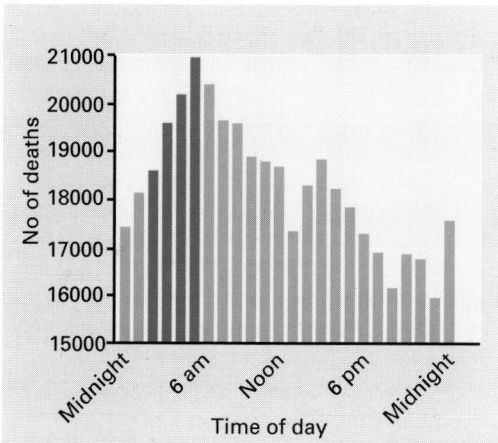

Circadian distribution of 437 511 deaths (from death certificate data).

Sleep disorders such as sleep apnoea, particularly when associated with other medical diseases, are associated with increased mortality. In a study of elderly women in nursing homes those with a respiratory disturbance index of over 50 survived only 17% as long as those with an index of less than 30, and all those with an index over 50 died at night.

Sleep related morbidity

Some changes during sleep that lead to increased morbidity
• Diminished hypercapnic and hypoxic drive
• Increased gastro-oesophageal reflux
• Onset of certain patterns of headache

In a random survey of 9003 British adults more variable sleep patterns were found among young (18-34) and older adults (over 65) as compared with middle aged adults. Particularly in these groups those sleeping a "normal" amount (7-9 hours) reported lower rates of illness.

There are pathophysiological changes during sleep which lead to increased morbidity (for example, hypercapnic and hypoxic drive is diminished, especially in REM sleep). For some patients, epilepsy is exclusively sleep related. Gastro-oesophageal reflux is more common at night. Certain patterns of headache, such as cluster headaches, have an onset during sleep.

One of the most common reasons for an elderly person to be placed in long term care is sleep disruption, which has an impact on caregivers that becomes intolerable. Many other sleep related disorders lead to admission to hospital, diminished productivity, and in several circumstances to more direct cost as a consequence of fatigue related accidents.

Impact and epidemiology of sleep disorders
Sleep and accidents

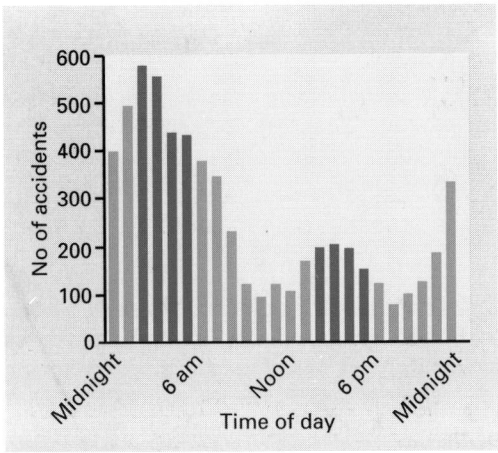

Circadian distribution of 6052 road traffic accidents judged to be fatigue related.

There is a peak of fatigue in the early hours of the morning and a second peak in the mid-afternoon. These peaks of fatigue are similar to peaks in the incidence of road traffic accidents that occur in a similar time distribution. Studies suggest that 20% of all drivers have fallen asleep behind the wheel at least once. One third of heavy trucking accidents which result in the driver being killed is attributed to fatigue. Studies in airline pilots with on board electroencephalographic recordings have documented sleep in some pilots while flying jets. Disruption of sleep pattern is thought to be a major factor.

Several studies have found a twofold to a sevenfold increase in road traffic accidents in patients with sleep apnoea. In one study, 60% of these patients described falling asleep at the wheel at least once while driving and a quarter falling asleep at the wheel at least once a week.

Sleepwalking not infrequently leads to accidents but occasionally leads to death, and rarely sleep related homicide is reported.

Financial impact of sleep deprivation and sleep disorders

> Studies have shown that insomnia is as powerful a predictor of early death as obesity

> Sleep disruption and sleep disorders have a profound effect on individual people and on society. An awareness of the specific disorders and their treatments is an essential part of modern medicine

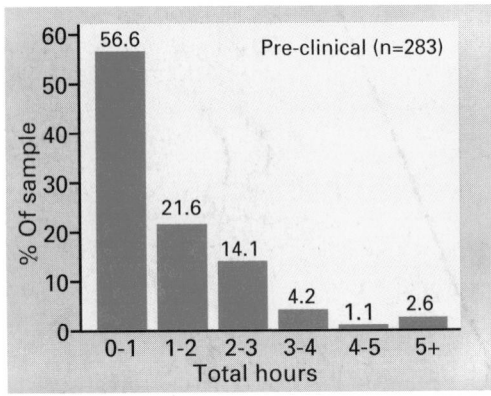

Currently medical students have little exposure to sleep disorders and the basic sciences underlying sleep medicine.

One estimation in the United States set the cost to society of sleep related problems as 16 000 million dollars annually. Loss of productivity as a consequence of shiftwork and the increased medical care of shiftworkers, admission to hospital of elderly people with sleep disruption, and the costs of accidents contribute in these calculations. Of this only a small fraction is spent on specific treatments and the training of medical staff. At present, the vast majority of patients with sleep disorders remain undiagnosed and untreated.

There are many other factors which can be considered in the broader issue of costs of sleep disorders. Several large studies have shown that insomnia is as powerful a predictor of early death as obesity. This implies both a human and financial cost associated with this sleep symptom.

The increase in work time (8% in the last quarter of a century) has had the consequence of reducing leisure time and sleep time. The consequence of this is fatigue and change in quality of life. These features are almost never evaluated in studies of wellbeing, although the diminution of both productivity and impaired performance (for example, among doctors working long hours or shift patterns) is increasingly documented. The erosion of sleep time in adolescents (almost 20% in this century) may have profound and long lasting impact on society if these adolescents are more sleepy and less able to learn.

Medical students receive very little training in sleep physiology and sleep disorders. In a recent survey of several hundred programmes, most pre-clinical programmes offered less than 1·1 hours of training in this area and 80% offered less than 1·1 hours on clinical sleep disorders.

The picture is reproduced with permission of the Mary Evans Picture Library.

FUNCTION OF SLEEP

C M Shapiro, M J Flanigan

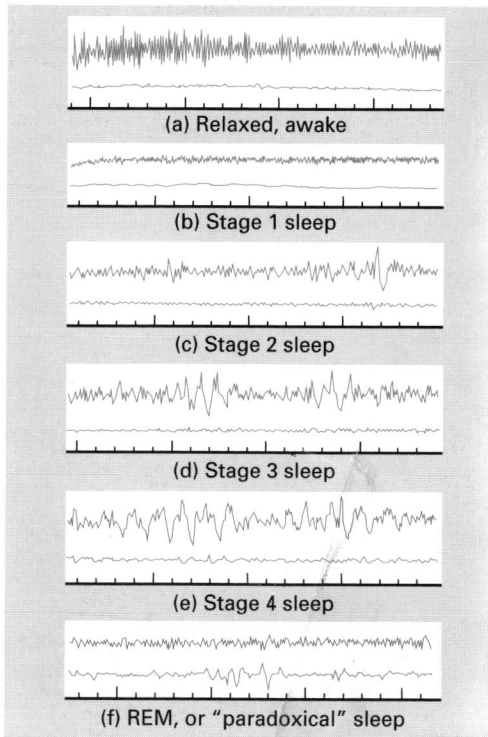

Electroencephalographs of a college student. The horizontal axis of each tracing is divided into units of one second. The top tracing is from one electrode on the scalp and the lower tracing indicates eye movements. Note the presence of slow waves in stages 3 and 4.

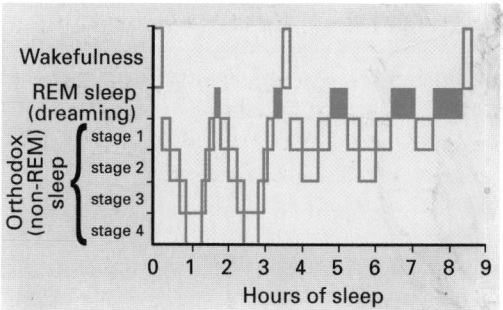

Cycles of REM and non-REM sleep. Each cycle lasts roughly 90 minutes; slow wave sleep predominates during the first third of the night and REM sleep during the last third.

Sleep comprises two distinct physiological states, as different from each other as each one is from wakefulness; they are known as rapid eye movement (REM) sleep and non-REM sleep.

Non-REM sleep is made up of four stages: stage 1 is a light, drowsy phase—the transition from wakefulness to sleep; stage 2 is the first unequivocal stage of sleep, with the appearance of sleep "spindles" and "K complexes" on the electroencephalogram; and stages 3 and 4 are known collectively as "slow wave sleep," or deep sleep, because of the emergence of low frequency, synchronised waves.

REM sleep is the stage during which most dreaming occurs. As people fall asleep they progress through the non-REM stages and then about 90 minutes later they have the first episode of REM sleep. There is a cycle of non-REM and REM sleep throughout the night, and as the night progresses the episodes of non-REM sleep become shorter, and those of REM sleep longer. Most slow wave sleep therefore occurs during the first third of the night, and most REM sleep during the last third.

Only during the past few decades has sleep been described in electrophysiological terms. As a result there has been a vast increase in the number of techniques that clinicians and research workers use to record and analyse the electrophysiological measurements of sleep. As knowledge about the physiology of sleep has increased, doctors have become aware of the variety of problems and abnormalities associated with sleep that are common among the general population, and so the discipline of sleep disorders has developed. Despite the wealth of information that is accumulating about the biochemistry and physiology of sleep, its precise nature and function are not known. A number of theories have been proposed, which include the hypotheses that sleep is needed: for consolidation of memory, for binocular vision, or as part of thermoregulatory evolution. In this chapter we deal with two of the more accepted theories. This explanation provides both a synthesis of relevant research, and background to subsequent articles that deal with details of the pathology of sleep.

Conservation of energy

> The metabolic rate is reduced at night, and particularly during sleep, by 5% to 25%

Most people's general activities increase during the day compared with the night. The concept of homoeostasis may be extended to explain that energy that is expended during the day must be balanced by a recuperative period. This forms the foundation of one of the theories of the function of sleep—that of conservation of energy. Expenditure of energy is measured mainly by the metabolic rate, which is raised during the day and reduced during the night (particularly during sleep) by between 5% and 25%.

Function of sleep

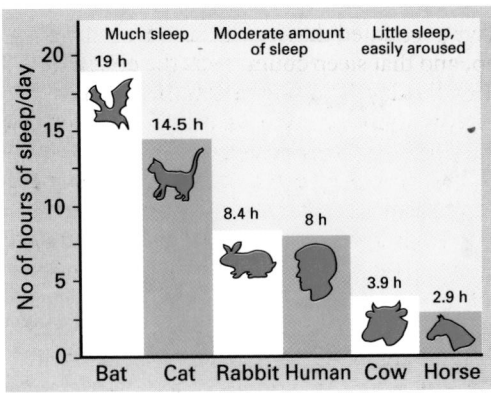

Number of hours of sleep/24 hours required by various animal species. Animals that are seldom attacked sleep a great deal; those in constant danger of attack sleep little.

Oxygen consumption, heart rate, and body temperature decline during the first few hours of sleep—the time particularly associated with slow wave sleep—and it is postulated that slow wave sleep is strongly associated with conservation of energy. There is a relationship across species between metabolic rate and sleep pattern, and there is evidence that people whose metabolic rates are high during the day have more slow wave sleep and sleep longer than people whose metabolic rates are lower.

Infants have the most slow wave sleep, and the amount declines with age (particularly stage 4 sleep). It has been suggested that this parallels the decline in cerebral and body metabolism that accompanies old age. High expenditure of energy during the day—for example, after sustained exercise in a fit person—is associated with both increased duration of sleep and increased slow wave sleep. Sleep deprivation is followed by increased amounts of slow wave sleep, perhaps as a consequence of the delayed drop in metabolic rate that normally accompanies sleep. People who sleep for a long time have high body temperatures during the day, and so their metabolic rates may be raised as well. In summary, therefore, the primary function of sleep may be to preserve energy.

Theories of restoration

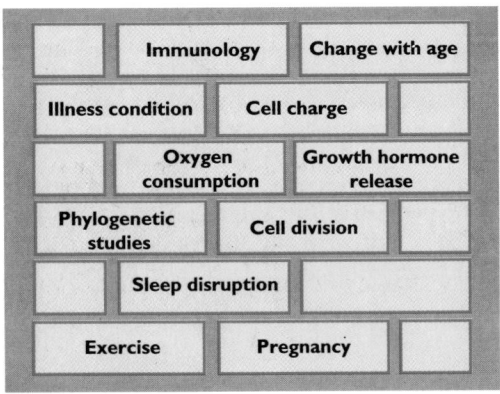

Types of research the results of which have built a "wall of evidence" to support the restorative theory of sleep.

The most widely held theory about the function of sleep is that it serves as a period of recuperation or restoration. There are two ways in which this hypothesis is interpreted: total body restoration and neurological restoration.

Total body restoration

The first hypothesis is that sleep is a process by which the whole body (including the central nervous system) may be restored. This theory is based on an accumulation of evidence rather than on a single critical observation. When the body is in a state of catabolism the consumption of oxygen increases. It is lower during sleep than wakefulness, and lowest during slow wave sleep. Paradoxically it is during this period of low oxygen consumption that anabolism is thought to take place. Low metabolic rates during sleep allow the net concentration of protein to increase as a result of both an increase in synthesis and a reduction in degradation. Though the processes of catabolism and anabolism are continuous, the relative rates vary according to whether the subject is awake or asleep, and it has been shown that the rate of anabolism is at its peak during sleep.

Growth hormone is released mainly at night, also in association with slow wave sleep. Direct measures of bone growth in adolescents show that sleep is associated with anabolism. Furthermore, treatment of short stature by growth hormone is more effective if the growth hormone is given at night rather than during the day.

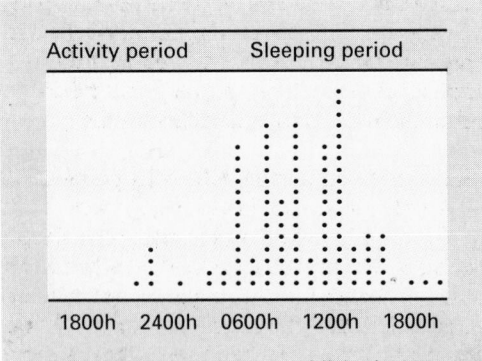

* Each dot represents a published report

In both diurnal and nocturnal animals the peak number of mitoses occurs at a time when sleep predominates in a wide variety of tissues.

Cell mitoses during sleep and wakefulness.

When the "need for growth" is great both the duration of slow wave sleep and the overall amount of sleep is increased—for example, during pregnancy, after exercise or loss of sleep, in hyperthyroidism, and during adolescence or the refeeding of patients with anorexia. Conversely, when less energy is expended—as in hypothyroidism—the amount of slow wave sleep is reduced. During periods of protein degradation ATP is consumed. If protein synthesis predominates over protein degradation during sleep ATP concentrations should increase, and this is indeed the case. These observations are supported by the finding across species that cell mitosis is at a peak during sleep.

There are several variations on the theme of total body restoration. It has been postulated that slow wave and REM sleep have different restorative functions, slow wave sleep being important for macromolecular synthesis and REM sleep for removing the synthetic products of slow wave sleep to maintain synaptic connections. It has also been suggested that during REM sleep neuronal connections in the catecholamine system are formed and that this activity is necessary to maintain cognitive function.

Brain restoration

Some research workers have postulated that it is the brain not the body that recuperates during sleep, and that sleep counteracts the effects of the metabolism of the brain during the day. They argue that the changes in physiological function that seem to accompany sleep may be interlinked, but are not exclusively interdependent. These scientists also claim that the exercise induced increase in slow wave sleep can be explained by an increase in brain temperature and metabolism, and after sleep deprivation it is psychological rather than physiological deficits that are most apparent. This emphasises that the restorative function is central rather than general.

One hypothesis is that there is a substance—"process S"—that accumulates in the brain during the day and declines exponentially with sleep. If, for example, after strenuous exercise (or under any condition during which the metabolic rate is raised) the concentration of process "S" is raised, then its decline from an initially higher level during sleep could account for the subsequent increase in the amount of slow wave sleep. Superimposed on this is a circadian influence called "process C," which is thought to play a part in the regulation of circadian body temperature and the length of sleep. Another theory is that the cycling of non-REM and REM sleep is fundamental to the restoration accomplished during sleep. Each sleep cycle results in partial restoration, and after a number of cycles recuperation is complete, which reduces the need for further slow wave sleep. This theory partly explains why the duration of periods of slow wave sleep reduces over the course of a night's sleep.

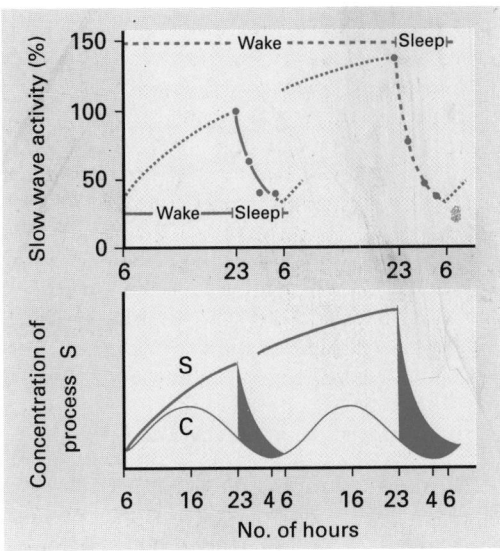

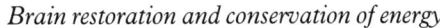

Time course of sleep processes after regular and extended periods of waking. Above: exponential decline in slow wave activity during four consecutive sleep cycles (value of first cycle 100%) for a baseline night (continuous line) and after sleep deprivation (dashed line). The exponential increase in propensity for slow wave sleep during time awake is indicated by the dotted line. Below: time course of process S and the negative function of process C.

Brain restoration and conservation of energy

One group of workers has put forward the idea that there are two systems of sleep that are initiated simultaneously and which together fulfil the requirements of both brain restoration and conservation of energy. The first system is known as "core sleep" and is thought specifically to restore the brain. During this type of sleep, slow wave sleep (particularly stage 4) and REM sleep repair and restore the effects of daytime cerebral "wear and tear." As the night progresses this core sleep declines, but the second system—"optional sleep"—continues. This promotes conservation of energy and is governed by the circadian and behavioural drive to sleep. This concept can be seen to be related to the theory of "process S" and "process C."

Conclusion

Useful addresses:

British Sleep Society
Department of Anaesthetics
Leicester General Hospital
Leicester LE5 4PW
Tel: 0533 584602

American Sleep Disorders Association
Sleep Laboratory
St Boniface Research Centre
351 Tache Avenue
Winnipeg
Manitoba R2H 2A6
Tel: 204 237 2760

European Sleep Research Society
IPM and Department for Stress Research
Karolinska Institute
Box 60205
S-10401 Stockholm
Sweden
Tel: 011 46 8 7286400

Australasian Sleep Association
Psychology Department
University of Melbourne
Parkville
Victoria 3052
Australia
Tel: 011 61 3 344 4000

In summary there are two main theories about the function of sleep—conservation of energy and restoration of energy—based on the drop in metabolic rate that occurs during sleep. There are several variations and subdivisions within the energy conservation theory; no one hypothesis completely explains the complexities and vagaries of sleep, but taken together they may form the foundation of the explanation for the indisputable need for sleep.

If sleep has a restorative function it is understandable why patients who do not sleep normally—for example, those with insomnia, medical disorders that disrupt sleep, or those who take drugs to alter their sleep pattern—may be more likely to develop psychiatric illnesses; why patients with hypersomnia have shorter life spans; and why patients with medical conditions that disrupt sleep complain that the effects of their condition are more profound and their quality of life is worse than those whose sleep is not disturbed.

The sources of the data presented are: Kalat JW, *Biological psychology*. 3rd ed. Wadsworth Publishing Company, 1988, for the electroencephalograms of the male student and the hours of sleep required by various animal species; Adam K, *et al*, *Clin Sci* 1983;**65**:561-7 for cell mitoses; and Borbely AA, in Kupfer DJ, *et al*, eds. *Biological rhythms and mental disorders*. New York: Guildford Press, 1988.

"I DON'T GET ENOUGH SLEEP, DOCTOR"

German E Berrios, Colin M Shapiro

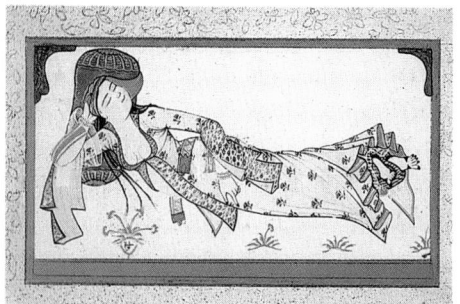

Eleventh century Turkish woman sleeping in her garden.

About a third of people who go to see their general practitioners and about two thirds of those who see psychiatrists complain that they are dissatisfied with the restorative quality of their sleep. Despite the size of these groups and the advances made by research workers, practical knowledge about the diagnosis and management of sleep related complaints is limited.

Patterns and habits of sleep are established in infancy, and core sleep variables (the proportions of stage 4 and rapid eye movement (REM) sleep), which are partly genetically controlled, enter a steady state by the late teens.

Sources of information

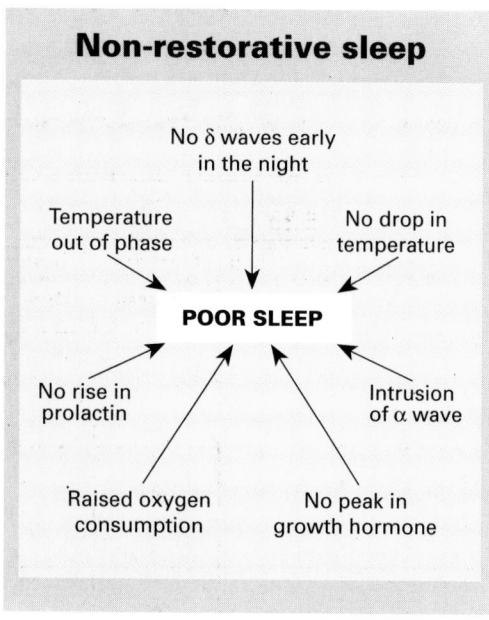

Non-restorative sleep

No δ waves early in the night

Temperature out of phase

No drop in temperature

POOR SLEEP

No rise in prolactin

Intrusion of α wave

Raised oxygen consumption

No peak in growth hormone

The complete assessment of sleep is based on information provided by the patient and relatives; on data obtained from polysomnography (synchronised recordings of electrical activity in the brain, muscles, and eyes); and on other physiological assessments—for example, breathing patterns and occasionally hormonal and biochemical estimations. Subjective and objective data are not invariably correlated. For example, complaints of poor sleep are not always confirmed in the laboratory, and major disorders of sleep architecture are often not accompanied by experiential complaints.

The doctor must therefore assume that feelings of satisfaction or otherwise with sleep are a final common pathway that combines neurobiological function with cultural and personal beliefs about the role of sleep, attitudes to life, life events, personality, and mood.

Many people with sleep disorders adapt, which may explain why the timing of a complaint may not be related to the sudden onset of a sleep disorder. In addition to whatever real or imagined sleep disorder they have, there is often a recent unrelated stressful incident that acts as the last straw.

Teaching about sleep disorders in most medical schools is inadequate, and many doctors have the same unsubstantiated beliefs about sleep problems as their patients. For example, many think that all sleep disorders are "secondary"—that is, epiphenomena of systemic diseases, psychiatric disorders, or psychological crises.

Complaints

> "Pseudoinsomnia" is more likely to cause poor quality sleep than a real alteration in the pattern of sleep

Patients often blame the quality of their sleep for any recently developed feelings of fatigue, depression, irritability, tension, sleepiness, lack of concentration, drowsiness, or muscular aches. The doctor must, therefore, find out whether any real change in the pattern of sleep has taken place; often none has, but patients who experience any of the symptoms listed above still ask "What else is wrong?" The doctor should widen his or her search for an explanation because depression, physical disease, hypochondria, and phobic states (that cause "pseudoinsomnia") are as likely to cause these complaints as a real alteration in the pattern of sleep. To presume pseudoinsomnia (or dysomnia) in the absence of other clearly defined illness is a mistake. There are various reasons why people claim that they sleep badly.

Even when a patient reports clear changes in patterns of sleep, they should not be regarded as the specific cause of coexistent fatigue or irritability. Indeed, the symptoms and the sleep disorder may result from a common cause (for example, depression) or they may be unrelated. In depression, tiredness and irritability may be accompanied by insomnia, or normal sleep, or even excessive sleep. The separation of fatigue, sleepiness, and tiredness in the context of insomnia is relevant but often difficult.

Changes in sleep habits should alert doctors to the possibility of a sleep disorder. The patient should be asked to keep a sleep diary. Information from a partner who shares the bedroom is an important component of a sleep assessment. The doctor should ask the partner about abnormal movements (including violent behaviour), snoring, and breathing noises during sleep. Changes in the pattern of sleep that must always be recorded include variations in the total time spent asleep; the time taken to get to sleep after the light has been put out; and mental activity and excessive brooding, anxious or repetitive thoughts, or panic attacks while waiting to go to sleep. The number and duration of awakenings during the night, and sensations just before and during sleep (for example, sweating, feeling hot, pins and needles, restless legs, and jerking) should be recorded. The affective quality of dreams (an increase in the number of anxious dreams and nightmares) may be a useful guide in patients with anxiety and depression. Alterations in diet, weight, lifestyle, alcohol intake, sexual habits, menstruation, and consumption of sleeping pills, "sleeping aids" bought over the counter, and other drugs should also be recorded, as these could disrupt sleep.

The results of one study showed that the average general practitioner asks less than three questions about insomnia before planning treatment, whereas there are many specific questions that should be asked about the onset of sleep, the length of sleep, and the patient's daytime performance.

Questions for partner who shares the bedroom

1 Does your partner stop breathing during the night? (Does this happen every night? How often does it happen?)
2 Does your partner snore, gasp, or make choking sounds during the night? (Does this happen every night? How often does it happen?)
3 Do your partner's legs twitch, jerk, or kick during the night? (Does this happen every night? How often does it happen?)
4 Have you noticed any recent changes in your partner's mood or emotional state?
5 Has your partner's consumption of alcohol, nicotine, caffeine, or other drugs changed recently?
6 What do you think is the cause of your partner's difficulty in sleeping?

SLEEP DIARY

Name: _____

Remember to complete this diary each morning approximately 15-20 minutes after awakening. Use the scale: −2=bad 0=neutral +2=good.

Fill in date under each day: LAST NIGHT: THIS MORNING:

	I went to sleep last night I felt (circle one)	I went to bed at: (time)	I fell asleep in: (minutes)	During the night, I awoke at: (time)	And stayed awake for: (minutes)	During the night I awoke at: (time)	I slept a total of: (hours)	When I got up this morning, I felt: (circle one)	Overall, my sleep last night was: (circle one)	I use an alarm (yes/no)
Monday	−2 −1 0 +1 +2			− − − − − −	− − − − − −			−2 −1 0 +1 +2	−2 −1 0 +1 +2	
Tuesday	−2 −1 0 +1 +2			− − − − − −	− − − − − −			−2 −1 0 +1 +2	−2 −1 0 +1 +2	
Wednesday	−2 −1 0 +1 +2			− − − − − −	− − − − − −			−2 −1 0 +1 +2	−2 −1 0 +1 +2	
Thursday	−2 −1 0 +1 +2			− − − − − −	− − − − − −			−2 −1 0 +1 +2	−2 −1 0 +1 +2	
Friday	−2 −1 0 +1 +2			− − − − − −	− − − − − −			−2 −1 0 +1 +2	−2 −1 0 +1 +2	
Saturday	−2 −1 0 +1 +2			− − − − − −	− − − − − −			−2 −1 0 +1 +2	−2 −1 0 +1 +2	
Sunday	−2 −1 0 +1 +2			− − −	− − −			−2 −1 0 +1 +2	−2 −1 0 +1 +2	

"I don't get enough sleep, doctor"
Secondary insomnia

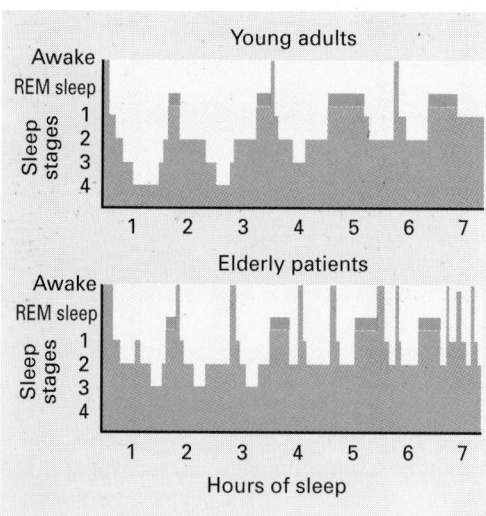

Differences in sleep architecture between younger and older patients.

Timing of insomnia

The timing of the sleep disturbance may indicate its cause

Primary insomnia

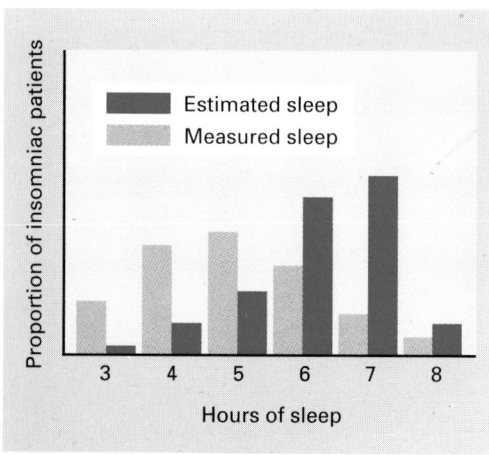

Measured duration of sleep among insomniac patients compared with patients' own estimates.

Among patients who present with a real change in sleep pattern, insomnia is the most common cause. This syndrome is defined as a relative lack of sleep, or inadequate quality of sleep, or both. The concepts of primary and secondary insomnia are helpful in clinical practice, though in some patients no distinction can be made.

Causes of secondary insomnia include psychiatric and physical disease, changes in shift work, drug misuse and withdrawal, personal crises, and changes in the system of behavioural cues and habits that encourage the onset of sleep.

Environmental changes (for example, moving house) that distort or attenuate established psychological triggers of sleep may cause insomnia. Changes in the temperature or lighting in the bedroom, environmental noises and smells, and the quality of the mattress and pillows may lead to disruptions of the initiation or maintenance of sleep. Using the bedroom for cooking, eating, studying, or watching television (as in a one room flat) may also cause insomnia in those whose sleep is fragile.

Transient disruptions of sleep (for example, those that accompany grief) may, in susceptible people, create feedback loops: inability to sleep for a few nights generates anticipatory anxiety, which in turn perpetuates the problem. This has been called "sleeplessness phobia" and triggers a habit that is referred to as "psychophysiological insomnia." It is often seen in people with panic disorders who fear that they might die in their sleep, and is common among patients who have had major traumatic experiences, in particular those who have undergone sexual abuse as children and who have come to think of the bedroom as a dangerous place.

Aging is also a cause of secondary insomnia. Old age can dismantle the architecture of sleep and is often accompanied by experiential changes.

Subjects may have difficulties with the initiation and maintenance of their sleep, or with early waking. For some daytime fatigue is the main complaint, but other causes may differentially affect the dimensions of sleep. For example, changes in diet, anxiety, sleeplessness phobia, high levels of arousal, obsessive thoughts, and environmental disturbances, may all disrupt the initiation of sleep.

Interruptions of sleep can also be random and cyclical. For example, random awakenings are caused by the sleep apnoea syndromes, coughing, breathlessness, and nocturia. Cyclical awakenings are more common in association with nightmares, migraine, nocturnal asthma, and pain from peptic ulceration (all related to REM sleep) as well as seizures (that may affect stage 4 sleep). Waking early in the morning often occurs in depressive illnesses, and daytime fatigue is common among patients with fibromyalgia, alcohol dependence, sleep apnoea, or nocturnal myoclonus.

Some subjects have insomnia despite the fact that little or nothing has changed in their mental state, circumstances, or environment. These patients should be referred to specialised centres where polysomnography may be carried out. In up to half of all patients who are investigated for insomnia, contributory information is provided by polysomnography.

If these facilities are not available the doctor must try to uncover further features so that the correct management may be undertaken. For example, it is useful to ask under what circumstances the patient is able to sleep. Some say that it is easier to sleep in noisy environments, and we have seen patients who can sleep only when listening to music through Walkman type earphones. Others can sleep only if there is absolute quiet, and if they start relaxing early in the evening. These two groups also differ in other ways. Those who require noisy environments are little affected (sometimes even helped) by drinking coffee before they go to bed. More surprisingly, they often state that in their earlier years they were the only ones who fell asleep when they took amphetamines during examinations. Those who require absolute silence are the opposite, however, and drinking coffee late in the day will disrupt their sleep. They often benefit from hypnotics such as benzodiazepines. It is unclear whether research will find some way to differentiate between these two hypothetical groups, or whether their behaviour reflects a difference in level of arousal. Their empirical separation, however, might prevent mistreatment, particularly when no specialised help is available.

Conclusion

Primary insomnia is rare

- Patients may need long term treatment with hypnotic drugs

Secondary insomnia is more common

- Treat the underlying cause:
  Psychiatric disturbance
  Physical disease
  Chronic pain
  Misuse of substances, particularly alcohol

Complaints of not getting enough sleep are not always related to actual or easily detected changes in patterns of sleep. Satisfaction with sleep is controlled by a number of factors and often is not associated with objective findings. Insomnia is the most common disturbance of sleep, and accompanies several diseases. Psychiatric and physical disease, chronic pain, and misuse of substances (particularly alcohol) are common causes of secondary insomnia. Primary insomnia, supposedly caused by dysfunction of the sleep mechanisms in the brain, is uncommon but may develop at any age and is occasionally precipitated by changes in the system of behavioural cues or contingencies that control sleep. Subjects with primary insomnia can crudely be separated into those with high or low levels of arousal. The diagnosis of insomnia must be based on a full history, clinical examination, and an understanding both of the patient's personality and environment. For this minority of patients long term treatment with hypnotic drugs may be appropriate.

PRACTICAL MANAGEMENT OF INSOMNIA: BEHAVIOURAL AND COGNITIVE TECHNIQUES

Colin A Espie

Presenting characteristics of chronic insomnia

Sleep pattern
Delayed sleep onset
Insufficient sleep time
Frequent or prolonged awakenings
Night to night variability in pattern

Sleep quality
Anxious or agitated before and during sleep
Feeling unrefreshed and unrested after sleep
Sleep experiences negative and not enjoyable

Daytime correlates
Sleepy or fatigued
Poor concentration
Poor problem solving
Tense, irritable

Insomnia is something to do with "not getting enough proper sleep." The essence of the definition is subjective dissatisfaction. Such concern may reflect a poor sleep pattern, poor quality of sleep, daytime effects, or a combination of these.

Effective practical management of insomnia must respond to the presenting characteristics of the complaint, otherwise they may persist. This article deals with the psychological strategies that have been systematically evaluated as potentially useful treatments of insomnia. They may be effective alternatives to hypnotic drugs, particularly in people with long term insomnia.

Non-specific treatment

Sleep education

Sleep stages and phases
Sleep is not a unitary phenomenon. Non-REM and REM sleep phases occur cyclically. Stages 3 and 4 of sleep are most restorative

Sleep functions and effects
Sleep helps the body recuperate. The brain is active in processing and storing information during sleep. Sleep is a natural process that will find its own equilibrium

Sleep developmental changes
Increasing age brings change to stage structure. It is usual to experience less "deep sleep" (stages 3 and 4) and more "light sleep" (stages 1 and 2) and more arousals in later adulthood

---

Basic education about sleep—Giving accurate information is a form of treatment. Although patients with insomnia are probably no less informed about sleep than good sleepers, there is benefit in discussing some simple facts and relating them to the problem. This will help the patient to place the sleep problem in its context.

Sleep hygiene

Exercise—Late afternoon or early evening is best. Avoid exercise near bedtime. Fit people have better quality sleep

Diet—Snacks before bedtime should be light and fluid intake limited. Best to maintain a routine

Caffeine—Coffee, tea, and "cola" contain this; intake should be moderated

Alcohol—Regular use as an hypnotic disrupts sleep pattern; a hot milky drink is preferable

Environment—Bed and mattress should be comfortable. Room temperature should be around 18°C (65°F). People usually adapt to noise unless it is acutely intrusive

---

Sleep hygiene—this term refers to general advice that may help to promote a good sleep pattern, though the elements themselves are unlikely to be sufficient treatment for long term insomnia.

Establishing an optimal sleep pattern

Establishing an optimal sleep pattern

(1) Go to bed only when you are "**sleepy tired**," not by convention or habit

(2) Set a **threshold time** after which you should monitor sleepiness. The difference between this time and waking time should equate to typical mean length of sleep

(3) Put the **light out** immediately you retire

(4) Do not read or watch television in bed; these are **waking** activities

(5) If you are not asleep within **20 minutes** get out of bed and sit and relax in another room until you are "sleepy tired" again

(6) **Repeat step (5)** as often as is required, and also if you have any long awakenings

(7) Set the alarm to the **same rising time** every day. This "anchor" should reflect your daytime/wake schedule

(8) **Do not nap** during the day

(9) **Do not take recovery sleep** to compensate for a previous bad night.

(10) Follow the programme rigidly for **several weeks** to establish an efficient and regular pattern

The sleep pattern is optimal when it is both efficient and regular. Sleep efficiency refers to the proportion of time spent asleep relative to the time spent in bed. Clearly, efficiency may be increased either by increasing the total time asleep or by reducing time spent in bed. Many patients with insomnia complain about difficulty in getting to sleep, or waking during the night, or both, and they often also wish to increase time asleep. The most reasonable first goal, therefore, may be to attempt to consolidate existing sleep into a continuous period and then permit duration of sleep to expand. Programmes designed to achieve optimal patterns have improved sleep efficiency considerably, and lead to rapid onset of sleep, greater continuity of sleep, and a more stable sleep pattern from night to night.

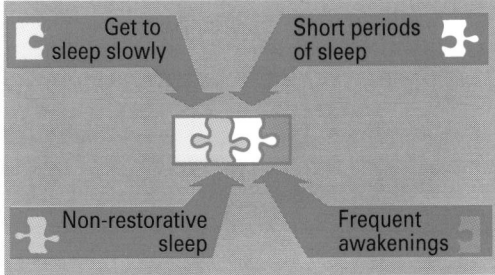

One classification of insomnia. (See page 8 for figure of non-restorative sleep.)

Much of the frustration and dissatisfaction experienced by insomniac patients is caused by the amount of night to night variability in sleep. The problem is not that it takes, say, 90 minutes to fall asleep every night; if that were so adjustment could quickly take place and anxiety would decrease. Rather it is where sleep is unpredictable that concern arises—when the patient does not know if tonight's sleep will be good or bad. The therapeutic goal is then to establish a regular, reliable 24 hour sleep/wake pattern.

Problems of tension

Dealing with tension and developing relaxation skills

(1) **Wind down** during the second half of the evening. The body requires rest as well as sleep

(2) Set a work/activity **deadline** 90 minutes before usual bedtime

(3) Practise a **relaxation routine** when in bed:
- Concentrate on breathing. Try to breath deeply and slowly. Rehearse subvocally "in" and "out" to respiration
- Tense and relax major voluntary muscle groups in turn interspersed with breathing exercises. Muscle groups comprise arms, neck, and shoulders; face and eyes; stomach and back; legs
- Take the exercises slowly. Do not overtense muscles. Relaxation is about "letting go"

(4) Practise the relaxation routine at other times during the day. Try to develop this as a **skill**

Many patients with insomnia report mounting anxiety and physical tension as bedtime approaches. A vicious circle develops whereby previous experiences of poor sleep lead to anticipation of problems and in turn to inhibition of relaxation (a necessary prologue to initiation of sleep) and to disruption of further sleep. Relaxation is incompatible with tension, so techniques that help tense insomniac patients to relax may therefore facilitate both onset and maintenance of sleep. In addition, and importantly, such patients may develop a coping response, which increases confidence in their self control. Relaxation should begin with the routine leading up to bedtime to facilitate the "wind down" process. A specific programme of relaxation exercises to release tension should be practised and applied during the first 20 minutes after going to bed, and at any other time of protracted awakening during the night.

Dealing with intrusive thoughts

It is more common for patients with insomnia to report problems with mental relaxation than with purely physical relaxation. Indeed, some report complete physical depletion but an alert mind, so cognitive intrusions must be considered separately.

It is easier to relax physically than mentally

Sometimes the thoughts revolve around daytime events and problems. Bedtime is often the first opportunity for rehearsal of the past day, for self evaluation, and for planning ahead to the next day and the future. Thinking things through in this way is not in itself pathological; it is in fact quite appropriate. It is the timing of the activity that is inappropriate and this may be related to an overstretched time schedule.

Practical management of insomnia: behavioural and cognitive techniques

Dealing with frustration or racing thoughts

(1) Do not try too hard to fall asleep

(2) State to yourself that "sleep will come when it is ready"; that "relaxing in bed is almost as good"

(3) Try to keep your eyes open in the darkened room and as they (naturally) try to close tell yourself to "resist that just for another few seconds." This procedure "tempts" sleep to take over

(4) Try to ignore irrelevant ideas and thoughts

(5) Visualise a pleasing scene or try repeating a semantically neutral word (such as "the") subvocally every few seconds

In other cases the content of the intrusive thoughts seems almost arbitrary. Incidental ideas come into the patient's mind, and partly because they are unimportant they cause considerable frustration. Another possibility is that the patient becomes preoccupied with sleep itself—or rather the lack of it—and about the potential consequences of another poor night's sleep on the next day. In these circumstances there is likelihood that a "performance anxiety" will be created—that is, failure to achieve sleep leads to added efforts to control it which are themselves inhibitory. It is not possible to make yourself fall asleep, and such efforts are best obviated.

General strategies for solving problems

Rehearsal and planning sessions

(1) Set aside 20 minutes in early evening, after your meal

(2) Sit in a quiet room. Have pencil and notebook to hand

(3) Treat this session as the pivotal point between day activities and evening time

(4) Reflect on the day past. Consider achievements in relation to objectives. Encourage yourself with achievements

(5) Consider problem areas and loose ends. Reallocate time to deal with these. Do not do the actual work. Note the decisions reached

(6) Consider also any other matters which may intrude on the sleep period—for example, emotional, financial, or other worries. Write down the first or next positive step of action to take and when you will take it

(7) If when in bed new thoughts intrude "refer" them on to next day

People who present with insomnia are often naturally mildly anxious. They may describe themselves as tense or as prone to worrying. Often they use their nervous energy in productive ways, but they may overdo it and cause stress.

Sleep cannot be expected to make up for an undisciplined or overly taxing daytime lifestyle; it is not infinitely flexible or restorative. Often such people will feel that they could cope better with work, responsibilities, and so on if their sleep improved. Too much is being expected of sleep; the source of the problem is being wrongly attributed. Some patients with insomnia, therefore, need to learn more about the practical management of time, people, and stress than about the management of sleep. Problems of concentration and decision making during the day may be attributable to a sleep disorder, but equally they may reflect work overload or anxiety. Irritability and other emotional reactions may have similar causes. The doctor's role in assessment is to help clarify the nature of the presenting problems. Insomnia can be a symptom as well as a cause of general difficulties.

Conclusion

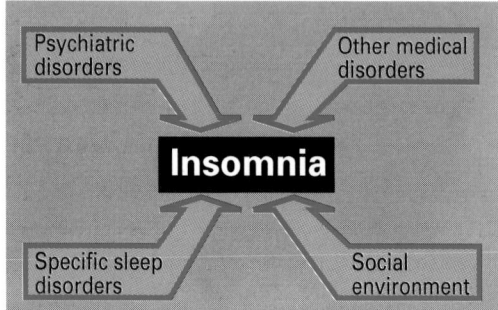

Pathophysiology of insomnia. The treatment should reflect the nature of the presenting complaint.

These cognitive and behavioural strategies should provide the general practitioner with non-pharmacological options for managing long term insomnia. Clearly the selection of treatment should reflect the nature of the presenting complaint. The evidence from our own and other studies of the outcome of treatment indicates that these strategies are effective when appropriately and consistently applied. As the goal of treatment for insomnia is often some form of change of habit, and the maintenance of that change, doctors must be prepared to direct and support patients' efforts to implement the advice given until satisfactory change is accomplished.

Further reading

Espie CA. *The psychological treatment of insomnia.* Chichester: John Wiley, 1991.

Lacks P. *Behavioural treatment for persistent insomnia.* New York: Pergamon Press, 1987.

Morgan K, Gledhill K. *Managing sleep and insomnia in the older person.* Oxford: Winslow Press, 1991.

DAYTIME SLEEPINESS

J D Parkes

Daytime sleepiness (hypersomnia) is a common and serious complaint, although it is less common than insomnia. In a recent community survey in the United States (in Newhaven, Baltimore, St Louis, Durham, and Los Angeles) 10·2% of the sample at the time of the interview described insomnia, and 3·2% described hypersomnia. Those most affected were young and unemployed people.

The complaint of excessive daytime sleepiness includes inappropriate and undesirable sleep during waking hours; reduced motor and cognitive performance; unavoidable napping; sometimes—but not always—an increase in total 24 hour sleep time; and occasionally states of incomplete arousal with automatic behaviour and sleep drunkenness, slurred speech, impaired motor control, and difficulty in focusing. The disability caused by severe daytime sleepiness is comparable with that of severe epilepsy. Many hypersomniac patients are labelled dull, lazy, workshy, or stupid, and if they need treatment are considered to be drug addicts. They have considerable problems at school, work, and home. Daytime sleepiness is an important cause of industrial and road traffic accidents. Gaps of several years between the start of symptoms and the achievement of a definite diagnosis of the cause of the sleepiness are common.

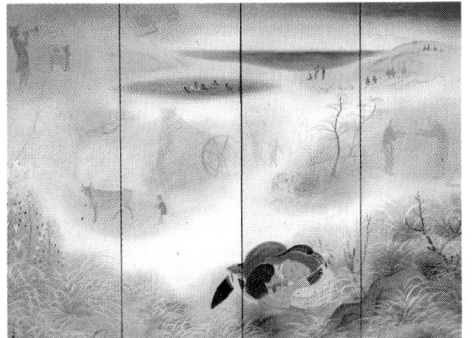

"Dream of the Home Country" by Shoko Kawasaki.

Excessive daytime sleepiness can be divided into two patterns: persistent—for example, narcolepsy and symptomatic sleep apnoea, and intermittent—for example menstrual hypersomnolence and the Kleine-Levin syndrome (both rare). This article focuses on the more common disorders.

When not secondary to persistent insomnia, daytime sleepiness usually has an organic rather than a psychological cause, though it may be an early (or the only) complaint in depression. Diagnosis usually depends more on history than on physical signs.

Patients' descriptions of tiredness and fatigue compared with sleepiness

"Physical" tiredness	"Mental" tiredness	Sleepiness
Tired	Poor concentration	Feel sleepy
Fatigued	Poor memory	Look sleepy
Exhausted	Little interest	Can't stay awake
Weak	Irritable	Sleep anywhere
Muscle aching	Jaded	Always half awake
No energy	Sad	Always dozing
Lie down to recover	Cannot get out of bed	Do not have to go to bed to sleep

History

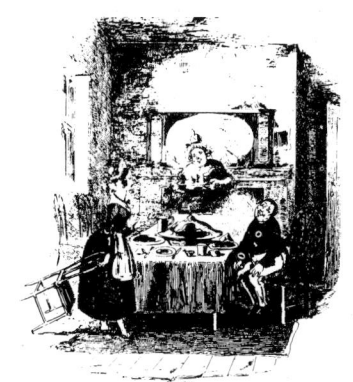

"Damn the boy, he's fallen asleep again." (Dickens.)

In many cases the cause of daytime sleepiness can be elicited from a careful history supplemented by watching the patient sleep. Important diagnostic features include episodes of sleep (rather than just sleepiness during the day); the inability to stay awake; and the propensity to go to sleep anywhere, not just in bed. Most subjects with excessive daytime sleepiness go to sleep readily at night (within seconds of going to bed), although their sleep may then be interrupted.

Fatigue, exhaustion, and tiredness are not the same as excessive daytime sleepiness and have different causes, and a difficulty in diagnosis is the fact that many illnesses and many drugs may cause both fatigue and sleepiness.

It is important to distinguish between daytime sleep attacks and other causes of altered awareness such as epilepsy, hypoglycaemia, orthostatic hypotension, cardiac disease, and various psychological problems. The distinction is usually obvious but, in particular, it can be difficult to differentiate between atonic seizures and cataplectic attacks.

Daytime sleepiness
Examination

Checklist to help define aetiological factors

1 **General**
Pain, weight, appetite, work, and environment

2 **Familial and genetic**
Some genetic disorders result in sleep apnoea (for example, nemaline myopathy and Prader-Willi syndrome)
Familial or genetic sleep/wake disorders include narcoleptic syndrome, sleep walking, delayed sleep phase syndrome, sleep paralysis, fatal familial insomnia, idiopathic hypersomnolence, and familial insomnia

3 **Neurological, psychiatric, and psychological**
These include depressive illness, Parkinson's disease, Alzheimer's disease, and high arousal with anxiety

4 **Metabolic**
Myxoedema and acromegaly can cause sleep apnoea

5 **Cyclical**
Includes menstrual nacrolepsy and Kleine-Levin syndrome

6 **Drug related**
Many drugs disrupt the sleep/wake cycle, particularly alcohol, sympathomimetic amines, β blockers, and hypnotics

In patients with the narcoleptic syndrome physical examination gives normal results. About two thirds of subjects with symptomatic obstructive sleep apnoea have signs of a restricted upper airway with receding chin, short neck, and obesity. Sometimes there are signs of acromegaly or thyroid disease. A third of subjects with myotonic dystrophy complain of extreme daytime drowsiness, probably from sleep apnoea, and in other neuromuscular disorders (particularly those that affect the diaphragm, such as acid maltase deficiency) there may be severe sleep apnoea. Autonomic failure in multiple system atrophy may present with obstructive sleep apnoea, and this is present in up to half of all children and adolescents with the Prader-Willi syndrome.

Investigation and diagnosis

Common causes of persistent daytime sleepiness

- *The narcoleptic syndrome*—This includes cataplexy as well as daytime sleepiness. Sleep paralysis, insomnia, and pre-sleep dreams are common
- *Symptomatic obstructive sleep apnoea*—This includes snoring, apnoea, and restlessness
- *Sleep related motor disorders*—These include hypnic jerks at onset of sleep, bruxism, and periodic leg jerks throughout sleep. Other parasomnias rarely cause daytime sleepiness
- *Depression*—20% of depressed subjects with a sleep disturbance have hypersomnia, not insomnia
- *Postviral fatigue syndrome*—Sleep, tiredness, and fatigue may be long term consequences of viral illnesses
- *Head injury*—Daytime sleepiness may persist for long periods after any head injury
- *Metabolic, toxic, and drug induced hypersomnolence*—The sleepiness of left ventricular failure, severe anaemia, and hypoglycaemia may result from reduced cerebral glucose oxidative metabolism. Alcohol, benzodiazepines, and other drugs may cause daytime sleepiness and a urinary drug screen may indicate the correct diagnosis
- *Essential hypersomnolence*—Some patients have recurrent daytime sleepiness, long unrefreshing naps, no sleep attacks, prolonged night sleep, difficulty in waking up in the morning but not cataplexy, sleep paralysis, or sleep apnoea. Total 24 hour sleep time is prolonged
- *Elderly patients*—Daytime sleepiness is common among elderly patients, and may indicate the development of circadian as well as sleep/wake disorders in degenerative brain disease. Chronic insomnia as a result of physical or psychiatric illness is an important cause of secondary daytime sleepiness

The history is more important than sleep laboratory investigations, but laboratory studies are sometimes essential. There is no one simple physiological measure of excessive daytime sleepiness, and for accurate assessment a battery of tests including subjective rating scales (such as the Epworth sleepiness scale), tests of sustained attention, and tests of motor and cognitive performance are needed. The best clinical laboratory measure of excessive sleepiness is the multiple sleep latency test. The test measures the "latency" (in a 20 minute window) to stage 1, stage 2, or rapid eye movement (REM) sleep on five occasions at two hourly intervals during the day under standard conditions. For reliable results the duration of sleep during the previous night must be known, and the patient must abstain from drugs, alcohol, and coffee before the test. A "median latency" of less than seven minutes on three or more tests is considered abnormal, but a few apparently normal subjects do fail the test (see p 34).

In normal subjects the first period of REM sleep during night sleep occurs about 90 minutes after the onset of sleep. In most cases the finding of REM sleep at onset of sleep during 24 hour sleep/wake monitoring, night polysomnography (electroencephalography, electromyography, and electro-oculography), or during the multiple sleep latency test supports the clinical diagnosis of the narcoleptic syndrome. A single day sleep recording without REM sleep does not exclude this diagnosis. In addition to or separate from the test, night oximetry or polysomnography may be necessary to define and evaluate hypersomnia, particularly when this is the result of sleep apnoea.

The three common causes of excessive daytime sleepiness are obstructive sleep apnoea (see chapters on sleep apnoea), the narcoleptic syndrome, and idiopathic hypersomnia.

The narcoleptic syndrome

The narcoleptic syndrome is characterised by excessive sleep and sleep episodes, and cataplexy with or without sleep paralysis, hypnagogic hallucinations (pre-sleep dreams), and disturbed night sleep. An unequivocal history of cataplexy is necessary for a definitive diagnosis.

Cataplexy (loss of muscle tone and paralysis of voluntary muscles) is caused by a sudden increase in arousal after being startled, surprised, or excited, and it accompanies many sporting activities, emotion, and in particular laughter. In contrast with agoraphobia and paralysis with fright in which the muscle tone is increased, in cataplexy tone in facial, postural, and limb muscles is lost and it resembles the physiological muscle atonia and paralysis of REM sleep although the subject is awake. There are small phasic movements during cataplexy, which are similar to those of REM sleep, with eye jerks and muscle twitches of the face and limbs, and are a useful diagnostic feature. Pre-sleep dreams and sleep paralysis also result from REM activity at the onset of sleep.

The usual age of onset of excessive sleepiness and cataplexy in the narcoleptic syndrome is late adolescence, with a range of 4-70 years. Roughly 5% to 10% of patients have an affected first degree relative (parent, sibling, or child). This syndrome has the highest reported HLA association, 98% of subjects having HLA DR2(15)/DQwl(6). Negative HLA DR2 typing largely excludes a positive diagnosis, but only 1 in 500 HLA DR2 positive subjects have the syndrome.

Checklist to help categorise the sleep/wake problem

1 Bedtime
2 Sleep onset time
3 Wake time
4 Get up time
5 Owl or lark?—What is peak time of waking performance and alertness?
6 Arousals from sleep—If yes, what time, how many, why?
7 Sleep quality (rate from extremely poor to excellent)
8 Excessive daytime sleepiness—If yes, what time, how severe, under what circumstances?
9 Sleep related motor events:
    Sleep onset (hypnic) motor jerks?
    Increased motor activity during sleep including leg restlessness or kicking?
    Epilepsy?
    Sleep talking, bruxism, sleep walking?
10 Sleep-atonia related events:
    Sleep paralysis (at sleep onset or on waking)?
    Cataplexy (stimulus provoked paralysis and atonia during wakefulness—a clinical diagnostic feature of the narcoleptic syndrome)?
11 Sleep related autonomic events such as sweating, piloerection, tachycardia in night terrors
    Respiratory abnormality—?apnoea, other respiratory irregularity, choking
    Nocturnal enuresis
12 Sleep related cortical-subcortical activity
    Dream frequency
    Dream timing (sleep onset dreams, equivalent to sleep onset REM activity, may occur in depression, following sleep deprivation, or in the narcoleptic syndrome)
    There is loss of dreaming in brainstem diseases such as progressive supranuclear palsy

---

Hypersomnolence

Common hypersomnolence syndromes, usually with prolonged night sleep, unremarkable sleep architecture, non-REM sleep onset, and periodic daytime sleepiness without cataplexy or sleep apnoea, are listed in the box on p 16 giving the common causes of persistent daytime sleepiness.

Sleep, movement, and daytime drowsiness

A few movement disorders during sleep may be accompanied by daytime sleepiness. These include hypnic jerks at the onset of sleep, bruxism, and head banging, but these conditions do not usually result in subalertness while awake.

Rhythmic leg jerking periodically during sleep with contraction of the anterior tibial muscle is a common and usually benign disorder that increases in incidence with age. The condition may be familial, and often is associated with restlessness of the legs (akathisia) during the pre-sleep period. Many sleep disorders are accompanied by this type of leg movement which is sometimes associated with daytime drowsiness. The diagnosis is established by electromyographic sleep studies.

Periodic rhythmic leg jerking during sleep with contraction of the anterior tibial muscle is common and usually benign

---

Treatment

Summary of treatment strategies in the narcoleptic syndrome

When the diagnosis is established central nervous system stimulants may be given, which improve the quality of life, but treatment may have to be continued all the patient's life. Treatment depends on the availability of such drugs as dexamphetamine, methylphenidate, and mazindol (it is not a licenced indication). Individually titrated drug selection, dose, and timing are essential. The patient usually feels undertreated, but this avoids side effects and it is usually possible to compromise. The dose should not be increased unless tolerance develops. Tolerance may be treated by withdrawal of drugs for 10-14 days, or by 3-6 month rotations of drugs. Doses higher than dexamphetamine 60 mg/day, methylphenidate 100 mg/day, or mazindol 10 mg/day should be avoided and it should be possible to control narcolepsy with lower doses.

- Patients with narcolepsy and other hypersomnias are not lazy, bored, incapable drug addicts
- Treatment is just as necessary for them as it is for patients with diabetes or epilepsy

Daytime sleepiness

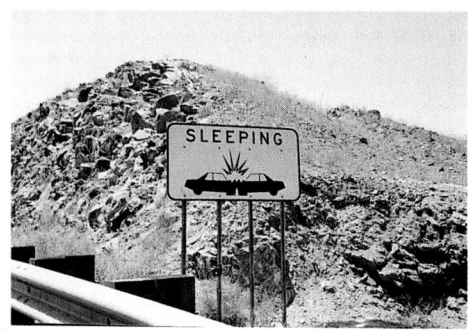

Sleep can kill.

Cataplexy requires separate treatment. Clomipramine 10-100 mg once daily is usually highly effective but the possibility of delayed ejaculation in men and increase in weight and appetite in both sexes must be considered.

If misuse of drugs is suspected, a plasma or urinary drug screen is indicated. Particular caution should be exercised when prescribing for young and elderly patients, and for those with personality disorders and bipolar depressive illnesses.

A simple sleep log with mood, alertness, and behavioural self rating scales during the first three months of treatment helps to monitor treatment. Changes in lifestyle and behaviour will also help.

For patients who wish to drive it is sensible to assess response over a six month period before considering issuing a provisional licence.

Central nervous system stimulants should not be prescribed to anybody with a history of psychosis, physical violence, or drug misuse, or to women who are pregnant or breast feeding. Cardiovascular risks should be assessed with care.

THE SLEEP APNOEA/HYPOPNOEA SYNDROME AND SNORING

N J Douglas

> **Failure to diagnose the sleep apnoea/hypopnoea syndrome leads to impairment of the quality of life and to avoidable deaths**

Awareness of the sleep apnoea/hypopnoea syndrome, which affects about 2% of the population, is increasing among both doctors and the public. It is readily treatable, and doctors should keep it in mind as failure to recognise it leads to serious impairment of the quality of life and to avoidable deaths. About 20% of the middle aged population are reported to snore each night, and this not only appreciably inconveniences their partners but also affects their own health and performance during the day.

Symptoms

Percentage of patients with various clinical features of the sleep apnoea/hypopnoea syndrome

● Loud snoring	95
● Daytime sleepiness	90
● Unrefreshing sleep	40
● Restless sleep	40
● Morning headache	30
● Nocturnal choking	30
● Reduced libido	20
● Morning drunkenness	5
● Ankle swelling	5
● Enuresis	2

Daytime sleepiness is the main symptom of the sleep apnoea/hypopnoea syndrome, and it may be serious enough to ruin patients' lives by making it impossible for them to work, drive, or even complete a conversation. In some cases the sleepiness results in road, occupational, or domestic accidents that may be fatal to them or to others.

Other common symptoms include unrefreshing and restless nocturnal sleep, nocturnal choking, feeling drunk in the morning and reduced libido. Nocturnal choking usually consists of patients waking up aware that they cannot inhale, which is an extremely alarming symptom that passes within seconds. Feeling drunk in the morning is uncommon, and consists of bizarre behaviour after waking up.

Spouses or partners should be interviewed whenever possible; they usually give a history of loud, intermittent snoring and most report frequent apnoeas, which is a useful though not diagnostic feature.

Most patients (85%) are men, and about half weigh at least 30% more than their ideal body weight. Obesity is thought to cause the syndrome by the fat in the neck squashing the upper airway. It is important to remember, however, that the syndrome can also occur in thin people. It occurs at all ages, but is most common in late middle age. In children it may cause failure to achieve at school and is often associated with enlarged tonsils.

Aetiology

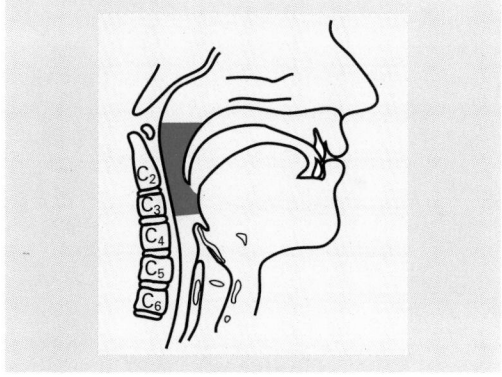

Site of airway narrowing in patients with the sleep apnoea/hypopnoea syndrome.

Apnoeas occur if the upper airway at the back of the throat is sucked closed when the patient breathes in during sleep. When the patient is awake the tendency for the airway to be sucked closed is overcome by the action of the opening muscles of the upper airway including the genioglossus and the palatal muscles, but sleep induces hypotonia and the upper airway narrows. In some the narrowing is not critical, but does result in turbulent flow in the narrowed segment which produces the noise of snoring. In others the airway may occlude (which results in apnoeas) or almost occlude (which results in hypopnoeas). These will continue until the subject is woken up, probably by the struggle to breathe against the blocked throat. The awakenings are so brief that the subjects are rarely aware of them, but they may be woken up to a thousand times a night and the disruption of sleep accounts for the symptoms of daytime sleepiness and impaired daytime performance.

The sleep apnoea/hypopnoea syndrome and snoring

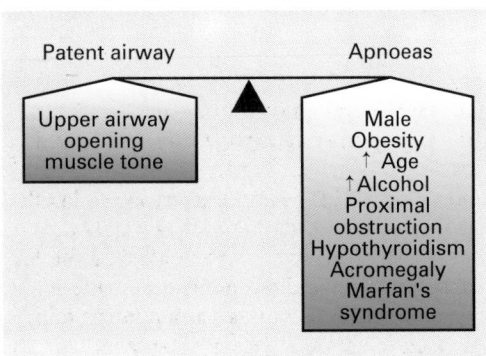

Right heart failure, secondary polycythaemia, and carbon dioxide retention occur rarely, and usually in those with underlying lung disease, as a result of the recurrent nocturnal hypoxaemia and hypoventilation. There is no evidence that sleep apnoea is more common among patients with lung disease, but when the conditions coexist the patients have two causes of nocturnal hypoxaemia and so the episodes are likely to be more common.

The sleep apnoea/hypopnoea syndrome is associated with an increase in mortality from cerebrovascular and cardiovascular causes. There is also accumulating evidence that people who snore habitually may be at increased risk of cardiovascular and cerebrovascular problems even if they have no other features of the syndrome. There is also evidence that some people who snore despite breathing normally during sleep have disturbed sleep patterns that result in daytime sleepiness and impaired performance.

Diagnosis

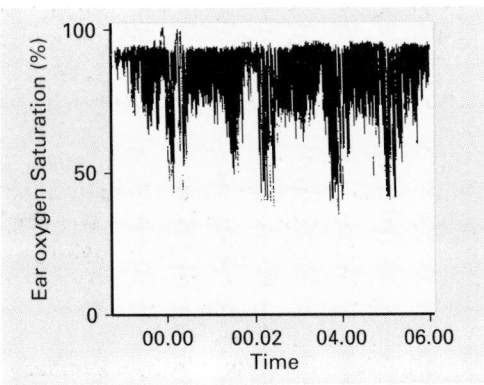

Oxygen saturation measured overnight by an ear oximeter in a patient with the sleep apnoea/hypopnoea syndrome.

Firm diagnosis of the sleep apnoea/hypopnoea syndrome cannot be made without overnight monitoring. In some countries, including the United Kingdom, doctors have tended to use the monitoring of overnight oxygen saturation as the initial screening test. Recent evidence indicates, however, that oximetry alone will detect only about two thirds of patients with the syndrome.

It is important that doctors who carry out overnight oximetry studies are adequately trained in the interpretation of the tracings, and realise that many patients who have severe sleep apnoea/hypopnoea syndrome have no disturbance whatsoever in their overnight oximetry tracing. The deterioration in daytime function in these patients correlates with the frequency of arousals rather than the extent of hypoxaemia. They should be aware of the potential pitfalls of false positive results whether in hypoxaemic patients or caused by artefacts on the machine.

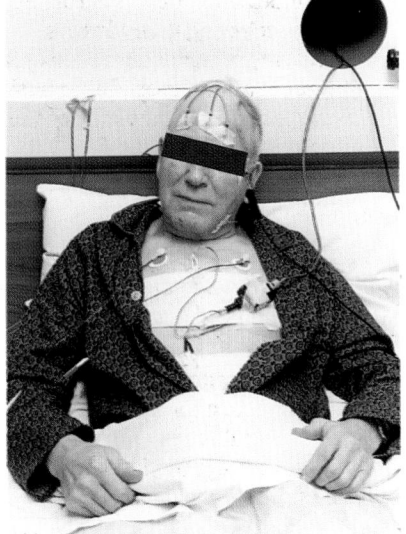

Patient wired up for a sleep study.

Another drawback of using oximetry alone is that it does not provide information about other causes of daytime sleepiness such as narcolepsy and periodic limb movement disorder. About half of all patients who undergo overnight oximetry alone for the diagnosis of sleep apnoea/hypopnoea syndrome will have negative or equivocal results, but their symptoms will be severe enough for a more detailed overnight study to be required. It may therefore be more convenient for more detailed investigations to be done in the first place.

The current "gold standard" for the diagnosis of the sleep apnoea/hypopnoea syndrome is polysomnography, in which the patterns of sleep and arousal are recorded by electroencephalography, electromyography, and electro-oculography; breathing patterns by semiquantitative recording of thoracoabdominal movements, oronasal flow and oximetry; together with electrocardiography and anterior tibial electromyography. The sleep apnoea/hypopnoea syndrome can be confidently diagnosed if there are more than 15 apnoeas or hypopnoeas in any one hour of sleep. These studies also permit assessment of the extent of disruption of sleep, irregularity of breathing, and extent of desaturation.

Differential diagnosis of excessive daytime sleepiness

- Sleep apnoea/hypopnoea syndrome
- Narcolepsy
- Nocturnal myoclonus
- Idiopathic hypersomnolence
- Psychological
- Drugs
- Sleep restriction

Polysomnography also enables the confident exclusion of the sleep apnoea/hypopnoea syndrome, the diagnosis of nocturnal myoclonus (which also causes daytime sleepiness) and, by the observation of rapid eye movement (REM) sleep soon after the onset of sleep, raises the possibility of narcolepsy. Narcolepsy may be difficult to diagnose, particularly when the sleepiness is not accompanied by any of the other features of narcolepsy such as cataplexy, sleep paralysis, or hypnogogic hallucinations. It is about one twentieth as common as the sleep apnoea/hypopnoea syndrome.

Treatment

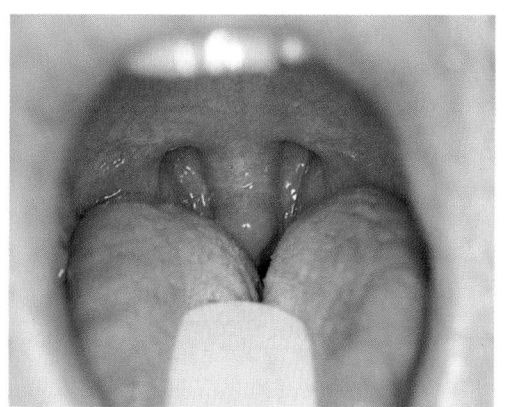

Enlarged tonsils and oedematous uvula in a patient with the sleep apnoea/hypopnoea syndrome.

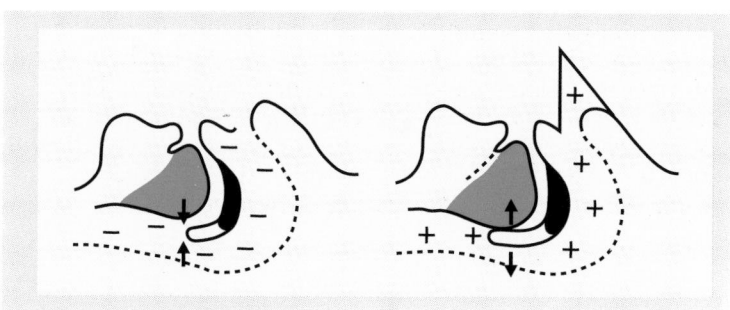

Diagram of pressure within the upper airway, during spontaneous inspiration, showing the tendency for the upper airway to narrow (left), and the effect of treatment with CPAP, which keeps the airway widely patent (right).

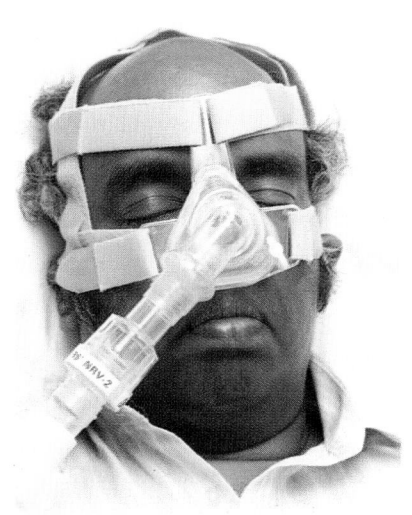

Patient being treated with CPAP.

Conservative

Obesity, enlarged tonsils, hypothyroidism, and acromegaly are all predisposing factors to both the sleep apnoea/hypopnoea syndrome and simple snoring and should be treated if possible. Patients should be encouraged to avoid alcohol and sedatives in the evening as these relax the dilating muscles of the upper airway. If those with simple snoring snore only when supine, the placing of a cork or a golf ball in a pocket stitched to the back of the pyjama jacket is a traditional and often effective remedy. Another way of dealing with simple snoring is to use a nasal dilating clip, which can be bought from pharmacies. This can become displaced, but in some cases it is useful.

Surgery

It may help to have the opinion of an otorhinolaryngologist in patients in whom the sleep apnoea/hypopnoea syndrome has been definitely diagnosed, to try and find out if there is any defect that is narrowing the nose or pharynx. Serious defects should be corrected, but operation on minor lesions such as septal deviation or nasal polyps is often unhelpful. Severe retrognathia should be corrected by combined advancement of the mandible and maxilla.

Operation in the absence of the need to remove specific defects has the attraction of being a single event, which will obviate the need for nightly treatment thereafter. At present, however, its role is both unclear and contentious. The operation most often done is uvulopalatopharyngoplasty, which is essentially a pharyngeal "rebore." Rates of improvement vary from 15% to 65%, probably depending on surgical technique and on selection of patients whose apnoea is the result of pharyngeal obstruction. About half of all patients with the sleep apnoea/hypopnoea syndrome obstruct at this level, the others occluding their airways behind the tongue. Unfortunately there is as yet no easy way of finding out the level of obstruction during sleep. If one becomes available, the ability to select patients better may make uvulopalatopharyngoplasty a more successful operation.

A serious problem with the operation is that patients in whom it fails may then be unable to benefit from continuous positive airway pressure (CPAP), because the pressure applied through the nose may leak out through the mouth as the seal between the soft palate and tongue has been destroyed and the CPAP will not blow open the upper airway at the site of obstruction. In addition, uvulopalatopharyngoplasty carries a certain operative mortality, and CPAP has been shown to decrease overall mortality.

Operations such as partial glossectomy, hyoidoplasty, partial mandibular advancement, and palatal laser treatment are still experimental.

Drugs

Drugs play no part in the treatment of the syndrome, because the side effects generally cause more trouble than relief of symptoms, and there is no evidence of reduction in either morbidity or mortality.

Continuous positive airway pressure

Most patients who fail to respond to the above measures should be treated by CPAP given through a nasal mask, which is tolerated by most patients. The pressure needed must be measured by a sleep study as too low a pressure may not only worsen the hypoxaemia but will result in failure to benefit, which may turn the patient against this potentially useful treatment. CPAP reverses symptoms rapidly and the change is dramatic, with many patients only then realising the extent of their previous disability. Side effects are few, the most common being nasal stuffiness.

The sleep apnoea/hypopnoea syndrome and snoring

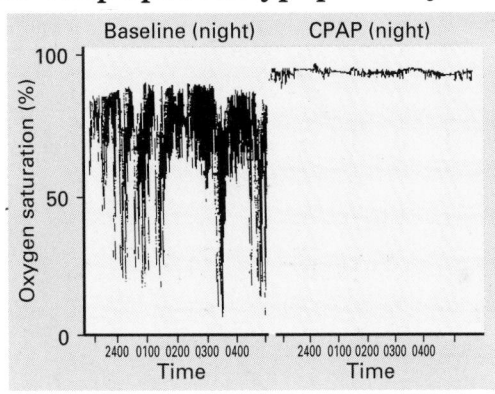

Overnight oxygen saturation traces in a patient with the sleep apnoea/hypopnoea syndrome. Left: Baseline tracing when the patient was receiving no treatment. Right: Tracing taken the next night during treatment with CPAP, showing abolition of episodes of desaturation by normalisation of the breathing pattern.

This often results from an air leak that develops through the mouth when the patient's muscle tone drops during sleep and can often be helped by the addition of a chin strap. If this fails intranasal steroids or atropinic drugs are often helpful. It is occasionally necessary to add a humidifier to the system.

The main drawback to CPAP is that patients need to use the machine every night of their lives, although this is a small price to pay for the benefit obtained. In practice most patients use the machine for about four hours a night, some use it for part of the night, and some occasionally omit it altogether.

Fewer than 1% of patients with sleep apnoea have apnoeas that do not respond to CPAP and result from cessation of respiratory effort—true central sleep apnoeas. Most of these have coexisting neurological diseases and are best treated either by intermittent positive pressure ventilation through a nasal mask or by diaphragmatic pacing.

Conclusion

> **Always ask:**
> - Do you fall asleep each day when not in bed?
> - Do you snore loudly and intermittently?

The main problem in the medical management of the sleep apnoea/hypopnoea syndrome is underawareness of the condition. Clinicians must bear the possibility of the diagnosis in mind and ask the appropriate questions routinely.

UNEXPECTED PRESENTATIONS OF SLEEP APNOEA: USE OF CPAP IN TREATMENT

T Douglas Bradley, Colin M Shapiro

Continuous positive airway pressure (CPAP) given through a nasal mask is standard treatment for obstructive sleep apnoea. By acting as a pneumatic splint and maintaining the patency of the upper airways during sleep it prevents occlusion of the airway and obstructive sleep apnoea, reverses associated hypoxia and hypercapnia, and so consolidates sleep. Because nocturnal gas exchange and the quality of sleep are improved the patients feel better, with less daytime sleepiness and fatigue. Nasal CPAP is well tolerated, and compliance is good.

The typical patient who needs CPAP has obstructive sleep apnoea and complains of snoring, restless sleep, headaches in the morning, and excessive daytime sleepiness. Occasionally, however, patients are referred for treatment of complaints apparently unrelated to sleep. They are seen by a doctor with a particular interest in sleep and sleep disorders, and as a result are found to have a sleep related disorder, the resolution of which cures the primary problem.

For example, some patients with impotence have been referred independently of that symptom for investigation of possible sleep apnoea. In some of those in whom sleep apnoea was confirmed, treatment with CPAP resulted in clear improvement in erectile functioning. Patients referred to obesity clinics who have undergone years of dieting without benefit have been investigated for sleep apnoea and treated with CPAP and have lost a great deal of weight. Treatment with CPAP may act as a catalyst to weight loss, and the sleep apnoea may then improve sufficiently to allow discontinuation of the CPAP.

To illustrate the scope of presentations of sleep apnoea and the success of treatment with nasal CPAP we present a series of case reports.

Confusion

A 61 year old man presented with a 10 year history of stable organic brain syndrome characterised by diffuse cerebral atrophy on computed tomography. The changes were most pronounced in the left frontal lobe and he had mild dysarthria and impaired memory.

He was admitted to the emergency department with a myocardial infarction after which he developed severe congestive heart failure with bilateral pleural effusions. He then developed acute confusion with complete dysarthria, outbursts of emotional distress, and faecal and urinary incontinence. These symptoms persisted for eight months, during which time he was in hospital awaiting transfer to a nursing home. He was in a vegetative state, unable to communicate, and incapable of doing anything for himself. He continued to have congestive heart failure despite aggressive treatment.

While he was in hospital it was noted that he had Cheyne-Stokes respiration when he was asleep, and this was confirmed by an overnight sleep study which showed recurrent central apnoeas with typical crescendo/decrescendo hyperpnoea alternating throughout sleep. These were associated with frequent arousals, severe hypoxia, and a complete absence of slow wave sleep.

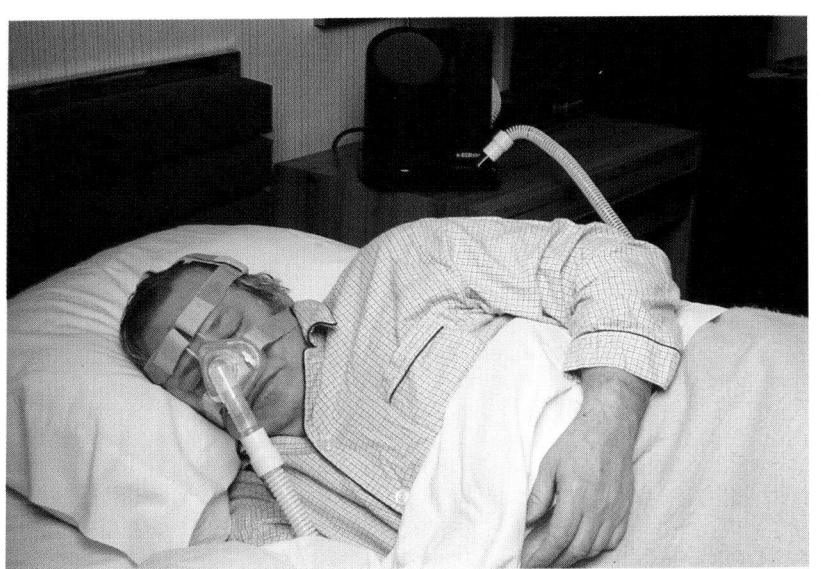

A patient being treated with CPAP.

Unexpected presentations of sleep apnoea: use of CPAP in treatment

We have previously shown that CPAP can reverse Cheyne-Stokes respiration, so he was given a therapeutic trial of nocturnal CPAP at a pressure of 10 cm H_2O. He tolerated this well, his Cheyne-Stokes respiration was reversed, and a repeat sleep study showed a pronounced reduction in the numbers of both apnoeas and arousals from sleep. The improvement was associated with consolidation of sleep and improved oxygenation. Shortly after starting CPAP he regained control of his bladder and his bowels. Within three weeks his pleural effusions had resolved and his dyspnoea had improved from class 4 to class 2 (New York Heart Association criteria). More importantly his mental function improved considerably; he regained his ability to speak, his emotional outbursts ceased, he became alert and communicative, and he had regained his previous state of health within a month of starting treatment. No changes in his drug treatment had been made during this period.

As a result he was able to return home. He has been followed up for two years, uses CPAP nightly, and has had no exacerbations of congestive failure or deterioration in his mental state.

Discussion

It is clear that Cheyne-Stokes respiration during sleep can give rise to the symptoms of sleep apnoea. In this case Cheyne-Stokes respiration probably played a part in the development of the demented state as well. Both cardiac failure and mental impairment were relieved by the improvement in oxygenation and the consolidation of sleep as a result of CPAP. This suggests that Cheyne-Stokes respiration or sleep apnoea should be considered in the differential diagnosis of acute and chronic confusional states.

"Heart failure"

A 51 year old man presented to the emergency department with acute congestive heart failure. He had been diagnosed as having idiopathic dilated cardiomyopathy and had had recurrent episodes of acute pulmonary oedema for two years. He was given standard medical treatment for the congestive failure, but continued to have mild pulmonary oedema and a resting left ventricular ejection fraction of 14%. He became short of breath after walking 30 m (100 feet) and had paroxysmal nocturnal dyspnoea.

It was noted during the clinical examination that he had Cheyne-Stokes respiration while sitting in bed, and during the apnoeic phase he would lose attention and fall asleep. He would then wake up at the height of hyperpnoea and would continue the conversation where he had stopped from the previous hyperpnoeic cycle. His wife said that he tended to sleep all day long and was never fully alert. She had also noted recurrent apnoeas, particularly when he was sleeping at night.

An overnight sleep study confirmed the presence of Cheyne-Stokes respiration with

---

- Sleep apnoea should be considered as a precipitating factor or in the differential diagnosis of:
  Confusional states
  Heart failure
  Nocturnal seizures
  Nocturnal bradycardia
- Cheyne-Stokes respiration during sleep can give rise to the symptoms of sleep apnoea
- CPAP not only reverses obstructive sleep apnoea but can reverse Cheyne-Stokes respiration as well

---

recurrent hypoxia and disruption of sleep, and he was started on nasal CPAP at night. This resulted in a pronounced reduction of Cheyne-Stokes respiration, much better sleep, and no more waking up with shortness of breath. His daytime sleepiness resolved completely. More importantly his exercise tolerance increased considerably, and he was able to walk several miles without becoming short of breath.

He was sent home taking nasal CPAP at night, and one month later his left ventricular ejection fraction had increased to 17%. A year later his exercise tolerance had continued to improve, he had had no further episodes of congestive cardiac failure, and his left ventricular ejection fraction was 22%. He was last seen after two years, when his medical treatment was unchanged. He had had no further episodes of cardiac failure, and he continued to use CPAP nightly.

Discussion

This case illustrates the importance of Cheyne-Stokes respiration in a patient whose main complaint was congestive cardiac failure. The respiration was associated with pronounced hypoxia and disruption of sleep, and reversal of the breathing disorder by CPAP resulted in consolidation of sleep and resolution of his symptoms of sleepiness and fatigue during the day. More importantly, his exercise tolerance and left ventricular ejection fraction both improved and he was free of heart failure.

CPAP does not merely reverse obstructive sleep apnoea, but can reverse Cheyne-Stokes respiration as well. In doing so CPAP can lead to consolidation of sleep and improvement of cardiac function.

"Seizure"

A 40 year old asthmatic man who was dependent on steroids presented to the emergency department having had a seizure during the night. He was obese, and weighed about 136 kg (300 pounds). A month before admission his asthma had worsened, his main complaints being orthopnoea and nocturnal dyspnoea, and he had increased his dose of steroid. A week before admission he had fallen asleep sitting in a chair while watching television

Unexpected presentations of sleep apnoea: use of CPAP in treatment

and his wife noticed that he had become cyanosed and then started twitching his limbs. He was unrousable, and developed tonic-clonic jerks that affected all his limbs before he woke up in a postictal state. On the night of admission he had had a similar episode.

Examination showed considerable obstruction to air flow, and he was treated with intravenous steroids and inhaled bronchodilators. Investigation for a seizure disorder showed no abnormality and he was not given anticonvulsant drugs.

It was discovered that he had a long history of snoring, was often sleepy during the day, and had headaches in the mornings, so he was investigated for sleep apnoea. The sleep study confirmed a mild degree of obstructive sleep apnoea that was confined almost entirely to rapid eye movement (REM) sleep and was associated with severe hypoxia and mild hypercapnia. Towards the end of the night, during non-REM sleep, the electroencephalogram registered several episodes of 3 cycle/second spike and wave seizure activity with no associated apnoeas.

His asthma was brought under control and he was started on nasal CPAP at night. His morning and daytime sleepiness resolved rapidly and he had no further seizures. A repeat sleep study showed that nasal CPAP had abolished his sleep apnoea and his oxygenation had improved. The seizure-like activity seen on the electroencephalogram was still present, but less frequent and prolonged than previously. He was seen after 14 months, when he was still using CPAP nightly, had had no further symptoms of sleep apnoea or seizures, and his asthma was under control.

Discussion

This case illustrates that there may be an association between nocturnal seizures and sleep apnoea but that it is not clear cut. The suggestion is that the combination of nocturnal hypoxaemia and disruption of sleep may have reduced the seizure threshold, and that seizures became apparent during the exacerbations of asthma and sleep apnoea. Proof of this is lacking, but the fact that he had no further seizures that we know of after reversal of the sleep apnoea is strong circumstantial evidence. It is also noteworthy that an electroencephalogram taken during the day showed no evidence of seizure activity,

though the one taken at night did. This suggests that patients with nocturnal seizures should have routine sleep electroencephalograms, and that sleep apnoea should be considered as a precipitating factor.

Pacemaker inserted—would CPAP have sufficed?

A 49 year old man was referred for investigation of possible sleep apnoea. In his letter the referring doctor wrote "Interestingly, five years ago he had a pacemaker placed for nocturnal bradyarrhythmias." The patient remembered being told that his heart had stopped beating for nine seconds during the night. In retrospect it is possible that he had had the typical bradycardia/tachycardia of sleep apnoea, but the clinical notes were not available.

At the time that he was referred he had many clinical features of sleep apnoea. The sleep study showed nine apnoeic events/hour of sleep, each one lasting from 16-160 seconds during REM sleep and 10-80 seconds during non-REM sleep. Oxygen saturation ranged from 78-97%, and 86-96%, during REM and non-REM sleep, respectively. The electrocardiogram showed intervals of paced rhythms lasting 10-15 seconds which corresponded with apnoeic events.

Treatment with CPAP shortened and reduced the number of apnoeic events, improved his oxygen saturation, and reduced the number of paced rhythms during the night.

Discussion

Cyclical bradycardia during sleep is a typical feature of sleep apnoea, and treatment of the apnoea would probably have obviated the need for a pacemaker.

Conclusion

The presentation of sleep apnoea is typical (see chapter on the sleep apnoea/hypopnoea syndrome), but there are times (particularly in women) when coexisting features mask the diagnosis. It was recently reported that about 8% of middle aged men and 4% of middle aged women are affected, and the diagnosis should be borne in mind when patients present with symptoms that may be triggered or exacerbated by sleep apnoea.

PARASOMNIAS

Helen S Driver, Colin M Shapiro

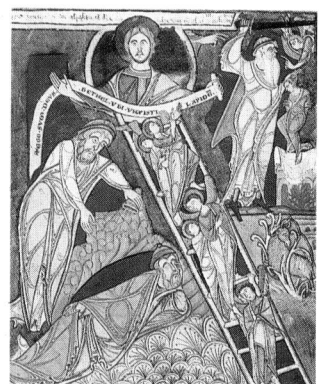

Jacob's dream (from the Lambert Bible)

Parasomnias are a group of acute, undesirable, episodic physical phenomena that usually occur during sleep, or are exaggerated by sleep. They are characterised by partial arousals before, during, or after the event even though they occur during different stages of sleep and at different times during the night. Most parasomnias are precipitated or perpetuated by stress, and an interaction between biological (often not identified) and psychological factors is presumed in many. There are three different types: those that occur during slow wave sleep, rapid eye movement (REM) sleep, and any phase of sleep.

Parasomnias during slow wave sleep

Features of sleep walking and night terrors

- They occur primarily in the first third of sleep when slow wave sleep is most prominent
- Slow wave sleep is deep sleep: it is difficult to wake the patient
- Patients rarely remember specific details of the event
- Conditions in which there are higher levels of slow wave sleep tend to increase the frequency of these parasomnias (for example, sleep deprivation, shift work, and alcohol consumption)
- Medical disorders associated with these parasomnias include obstructive sleep apnoea syndrome, migraine, and epileptic seizures
- They are more common in children (the onset is usually before the age of 10 years). Children have more slow wave sleep than adults
- One person may have more than one form of parasomnia. There may be a common genetic and neurophysiological substrate in somnambulism and night terrors
- These parasomnias may occur in response to stress or anxiety and may be more common when sleep schedules are irregular

---

Slow wave sleep is non-REM sleep (stages 3 and 4), when δ waves predominate on the electroencephalogram. Somnambulism (sleep walking) and night terrors ("pavor nocturnus" in children and "incubus" in adults) are in this group, and seem to be "disorders of arousal." Patients who are disturbed rather than becoming fully awake during slow wave sleep enter a state of confusion and disorientation. Such patients seem to have a generalised, hypersynchronous, symmetrical δ pattern on the electroencephalogram, which precedes the parasomnia and persists during it, and may be an indicator of disturbed sleep.

Both somnambulism and night terrors are described as "immaturities of the central nervous system" in children, but are thought to be more indicative of psychopathology in adults.

Differences between nightmares and night terrors

	Nightmare	Night terror
Sleep stage	REM sleep	Non-REM sleep
Timing	Late in sleeping period	Often during first hour after onset of sleep
Recall	Usual	Usually absent
Behaviour during event	Quickly in contact with surroundings	Often "out of reach"
Family pattern	Not confirmed	Yes
Treatment	Clomipramine, psychotherapy	Sleep hygiene, benzodiazepines

Sleep walking

Recent studies have suggested that adult sleep walkers may have a distinctive personality profile. During sleep walking vision seems to remain intact; coordination of the central nervous system is maintained to some extent, although accidental injuries have been reported. An episode can last from minutes to an hour. More than one episode a night is rare, as is the likelihood of complex manoeuvres.

Coping with night terrors: a guide for parents

Normal sleep includes cycles of light sleep, deep sleep, and partial waking. Occasionally dreams, nightmares, and night terrors can disturb a child's sleep.

What are night terrors?

Night terrors are brief episodes (about 10-20 minutes) of partial waking that occur during deep sleep and are accompanied by thrashing, kicking, rolling movements, and unintelligible speech. The child does not respond to voice, touch, or reassurance. They are most common among children aged 2-6 years and usually occur within the first two hours of going to sleep.

Important facts about night terrors

(1) The child will not remember it in the morning
(2) Trying to wake the child during the night terror rarely shortens it
(3) The child is not ill
(4) Night terrors do not have any long term ill effects
(5) They often occur only once a night, and not every night. Usually they will decrease and disappear three to four months after they start
(6) Overtiredness and changes in routine will make them worse

What parents can do

(1) Stay calm during the night terror
(2) Restrain the child physically only to prevent self injury
(3) Place anything breakable out of reach. If necessary lock doors and windows
(4) Maintain the child's routine as far as possible, and encourage periods of rest after physical activity
(5) Reassure siblings that the terrors will do no harm and will go away
(6) Remember that the child will have no memory of the incident the next day
(7) Your reaction and that of siblings may upset the child who is having the night terrors; reassure the child
(8) Try to find out if the child is worried about anything, and see if you can help
(9) Consult your doctor if the type and frequency of night terrors changes, or if they occur for more than three months

Many patients with severe sleep walking tell doctors at specialist clinics that they have previously been "fobbed off." This is clinical negligence. It is particularly important that these patients are instructed to sleep in a safe environment. There should be bars on upstairs windows; stair gates, locks (possibly combination locks) on outside doors; and they should request rooms on the ground floor in hotels. They should be advised to avoid sleep deprivation (long drives at night, or shift work) or other circumstances that might make them excessively sleepy—for example, drinking alcohol before going to bed. Psychotherapy may benefit some adult sleep walkers.

Night terrors

Night terrors usually start with a terrifying scream, increased heart and respiratory rates, sweating, possibly a penile erection, and a frightened expression. They last from one to several minutes, and should be distinguished from nightmares.

Psychotherapy should be the first line of treatment, particularly in children. Low doses of a benzodiazepine (for example, diazepam 2-10 mg before sleep) may help, but there is a high rate of relapse particularly at times of stress. A regular bedtime routine that permits sufficient sleep often leads to improvement in children. Many simple parasomnias improve with improved sleep hygiene, particularly decreased alcohol and caffeine consumption. Sleep eating is an unusual parasomnia that may have more psychological dimensions than other parasomnias.

Parasomnias during REM sleep

Parasomnias during REM sleep occur during the middle and last third of sleep, when REM periods are more abundant and intense; patients arouse easily and quickly.

Dream anxiety attacks

Dream anxiety attacks or nightmares are frightening dreams with vivid recall. Often a quick motor reaction in the nightmare is played out which wakes the patient up. These attacks typically start during the late teens and correlate with increases in stress, depression, painful life events, insecurity, anxiety, and guilt; they are common among patients with post-traumatic stress disorder. Others causes include fever; abrupt stopping of drugs that suppress REM sleep such as amphetamines, many antidepressants, and benzodiazepines (particularly those with short half lives); and acute alcohol detoxification. These lead to a rebound/recoil in REM sleep which promotes nightmares. Treatment is with drugs that suppress REM sleep (clomipramine is probably the most useful) and psychotherapy is occasionally beneficial. Children need support and comfort. Environmental factors such as horror films may be important triggers.

Comparison of sleep disorders in children

	Dreams	Nightmares	Sleepwalking	Night terrors
Sleep stage	Light non-REM and REM	REM	Stage 4 non-REM	Stage 4 non-REM sleep
Time after went to sleep (h)	3-6	3-6	1-2	1-2
Sounds	None	Occasional unintelligible sounds	Occasional meaningless speech	Scream± continuous loud meaningless speech
Motor movement	Little or none	Little until point of waking	Usually purposeful and unpredictable; child rarely stays in bed or room	Purposeless movement; child usually stays in bed
Response to parent	Awakes easily to stimuli	Awakes easily to stimuli; reorients in several minutes	Little to none	Little to none
Memory of event	Can describe immediately	Can describe immediately; often able to remember event following day	None	None

Parasomnias

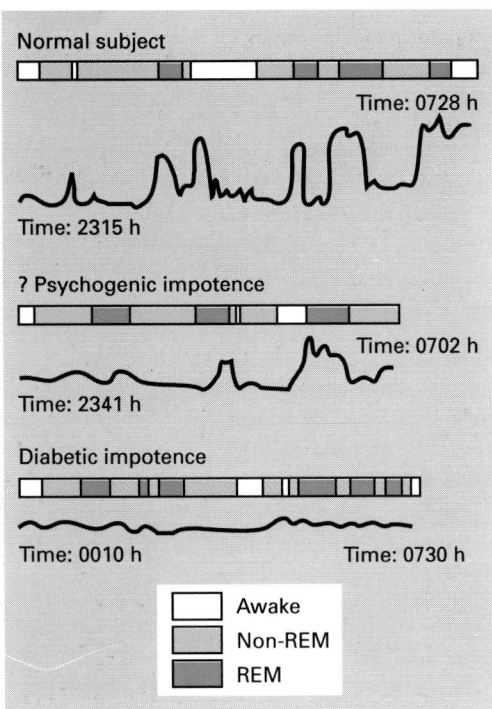

Normal subject

Time: 0728 h

Time: 2315 h

? Psychogenic impotence

Time: 0702 h

Time: 2341 h

Diabetic impotence

Time: 0010 h   Time: 0730 h

☐ Awake
▨ Non-REM
▨ REM

Tracings show strain gauge measurements of erectile function, which increases during REM sleep.

Sleep related cluster headaches and chronic paroxysmal hemicrania

These are vascular headaches that are associated with REM sleep; the sleeper often wakes up with agonising pain.

Sleep related asthma

There is a "morning dip" during which attacks of asthma are exacerbated and possibly triggered by REM sleep.

Impaired penile tumescence

Nocturnal erections are a normal component of REM sleep in men. Their occurrence can be used to distinguish organic from psychogenic impotence. In rare cases they become painful and arouse the sleeper.

Other parasomnias

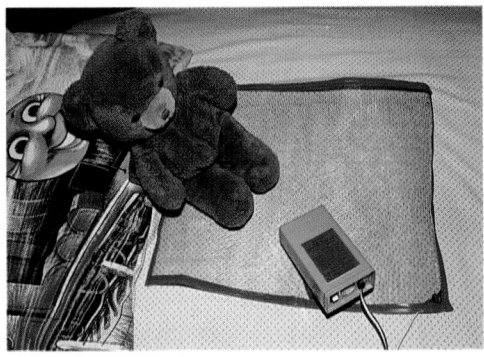

A child's pad and buzzer enuretic alarm. When the pad gets wet the buzzer sounds, waking the child.

Other parasomnias may occur during any phase of sleep, but particularly stages 1 and 2, and the transitional phases.

Enuresis (bed wetting)

Primary enuresis occurs in children in whom nocturnal toilet training has never been accomplished (between 3 and 6 years). Secondary enuresis occurs in those who have been toilet trained and stopped wetting the bed for at least a few months before starting to wet the bed again. It seems to occur in a random pattern throughout all stages of sleep and is sometimes thought to be related to an immature central nervous system. Sleep related enuresis occurs in about 1-3% of the adult population and in roughly 70% of mentally retarded patients. Genetic factors may be involved, and children with sleep related enuresis seem to have a higher incidence of sleep walking and of night terrors.

Explaining to patients with enuresis that they have different sleep patterns and do not always sense the need to urinate can help to relieve the shame and guilt that they feel. They can be treated with low doses of a tricyclic antidepressant such as imipramine; behavioural techniques such as the use of a pad and buzzer, bladder training, and fluid restriction at night can often eliminate the bed wetting. In difficult cases nocturnal antidiuretic hormone secretion should be considered.

Bruxism

Bruxism, or grinding the teeth, occurs mainly during sleep stages 1 and 2, and during partial arousals, and usually lasts for about 10 seconds. It comprises the forcible grinding or gnashing of the teeth by rhythmic contraction of the masseter and other muscles during sleep, usually without the patient being aware. The most common symptom is damage to the teeth and, in severe cases, facial pain. Diurnal or daytime bruxism is related to stress and can be treated by biofeedback. Nocturnal bruxism is common (from 5% to 20% of the population) and the aetiology is unknown. The usual "treatment" is a rubber mouthguard which is worn over the teeth at night.

Head banging

This describes the rhythmic rocking movements of the head or body which occur just before sleep or during stages 1 and 2. It is usually limited to childhood but may be seen in adults.

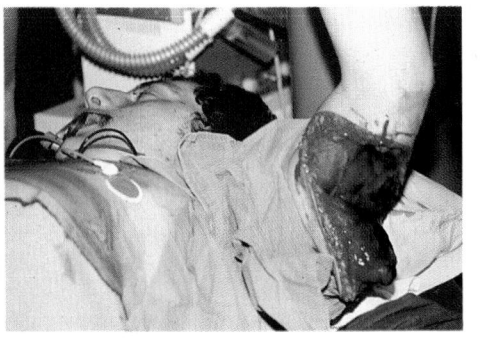

This patient walked through a plate glass door while asleep. His mother and daughter also walk in their sleep.

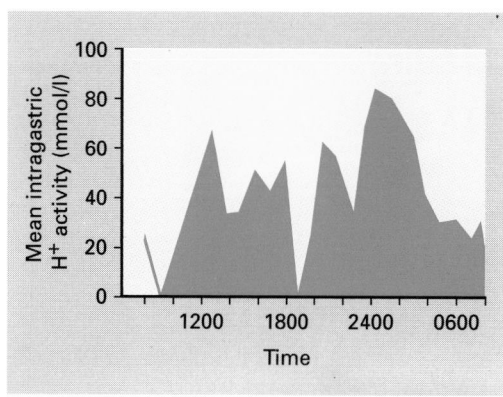

Diagram showing 24 hour gastic acid secretion in a patient with duodenal ulcer. There is a pronounced increase during the night.

Conclusion

| Parasomnias should be taken seriously |

Familial sleep paralysis

This is usually a symptom of narcolepsy, although a benign form may occur in isolation.

Cardiovascular symptoms

These may be related more to prolonged recumbence than to sleep. Some may be the result of the low systemic blood pressure during slow wave sleep or to the increased and highly variable heart rate and blood pressure associated with REM sleep.

Gastro-oesophageal reflux

This causes patients to wake with heartburn, or a feeling of general pain or tightness in the chest, or a sour taste in the mouth. The cause may be unusually low pressure at the lower oesophageal sphincter. The patient should sleep in a bed that is propped up at the top end, but weight loss and general medical treatment are also required. Reassurance about the distinction between oesophageal reflux and nocturnal angina is important.

Parasomnias can be alarming to the patient, parents (they occur more commonly in children), and bed partners. Rather than being treated with humour and then neglected, patients with a parasomnia and the family need reassurance, education, and treatment. This remains an understudied and underappreciated clinical area.

We thank Dr Alan M Jackson for taking the picture of the enuresis alarm.

CIRCADIAN RHYTHMS

Jim Waterhouse, David Minors

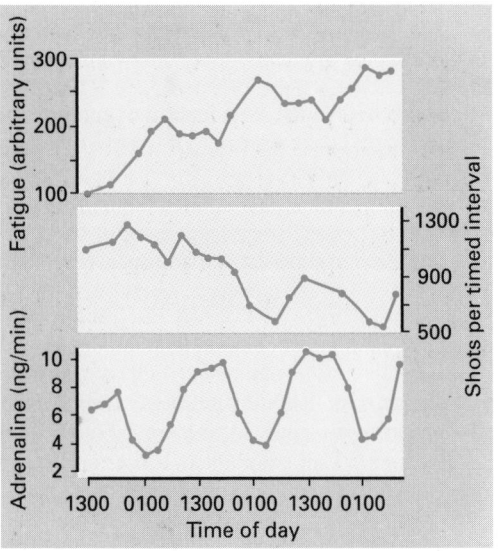

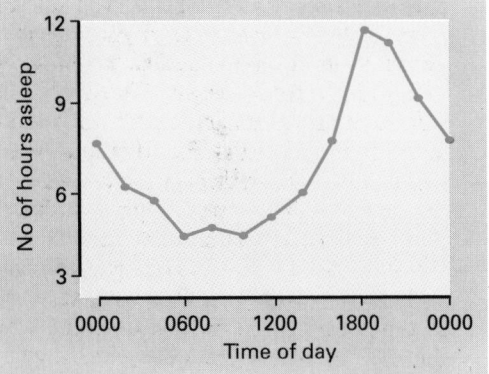

Three-hourly ratings of fatigue, speed of firing at a target (shots/timed interval), and urinary excretion of adrenaline in a group of soldiers who stayed awake for about three days in constant conditions.

Length of time that subjects could sleep in the uniform conditions of a sleep laboratory when they had started their sleep at different times of the day. Sleeps that started at the end of the night were short (despite the subjects not having been allowed to sleep that night) whereas those that started at about 1800 lasted much longer.

We do not feel tired only because we have been awake and active for several hours. If that were so our feelings of fatigue would increase inexorably and progressively during the time that had elapsed since our last sleep. Instead, when we stay up all night fatigue increases until it reaches a peak at about 0500, but then it decreases at least until the next evening. Superimposed on the general increase in fatigue there are daily cycles, each of which show a "fatigue maximum" in the middle of the normal time for sleep and a "fatigue minimum" in the late afternoon. Fatigue has a rhythmic component, therefore, and this is associated with rhythmic changes in our ability to fall asleep and to stay asleep.

Such rhythms are only a few of the many that permeate the physiology, psychology, and biochemistry of the individual. When several rhythms are considered those that are linked causally show characteristic and reliable phase relationships between each other. For example, in the case shown in the first figure, the rhythms of urinary adrenaline excretion and the speed of shooting at a target are in phase with each other and the rhythm of fatigue is always the inverse.

Body temperature

The length of sleep is also associated with body temperature and this can be usefully examined in free running experiments—that is, ones in which subjects are studied individually in an environment from which all external indicators of the passage of time have been excluded. In such conditions most subjects have synchronised rhythms and go to sleep just before their body temperature falls to its minimum. By contrast, in some, there is no synchronisation between the rhythms of body temperature and the sleep/wake cycle. As a result sleep is initiated at all phases of the temperature rhythm and this influences the length of sleep that is achieved. Almost identical results are obtained when volunteers attempt to sleep at different times of the day in a sleep laboratory. Because the temperature minimum occurs at about 0500 in people with a normal life style and sleeping about eight hours, there is considerable agreement between the results of free running experiments, laboratory studies, and common experience.

Sleep/wake rhythms

There is also an inverse relationship between the length of time spent awake and the duration of the subsequent period of sleep. This is more easily understood if sleep is seen as part of a sleep/wake rhythm in addition to a time of recuperation; going to bed late means that you will sooner reach a time for waking, and vice versa.

The constant association that normally exists between rhythms is biologically adaptive, so in the evening body temperature and plasma adrenaline concentration fall, we feel tired, and it is easy to have unbroken sleep. By contrast, even if we have been awake all night, it is difficult to have unbroken sleep starting at about 0800 because our rhythms of body temperature, adrenaline, and general alertness will all be on their rising phases.

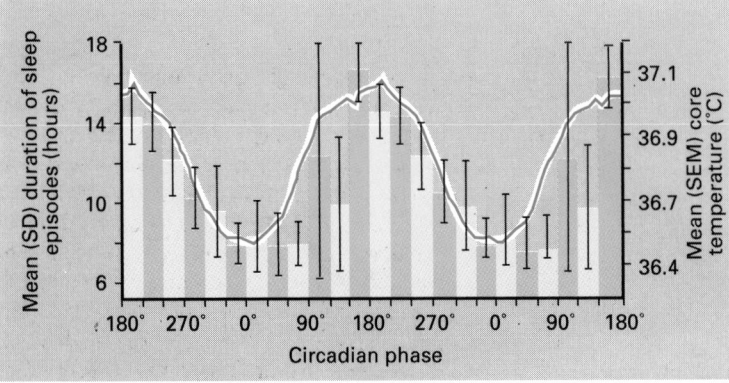

Mean core temperature and length of sleep in subjects in a time free environment whose sleep/wake and temperature cycles were not synchronised. Mean temperature is shown as solid line, and mean (SEM) length of sleep begun at that circadian phase of the temperature rhythm as bars. (360°=free running period of temperature rhythm (about 25 h), and 0°=minimum temperature.)

Loss of sleep and naps

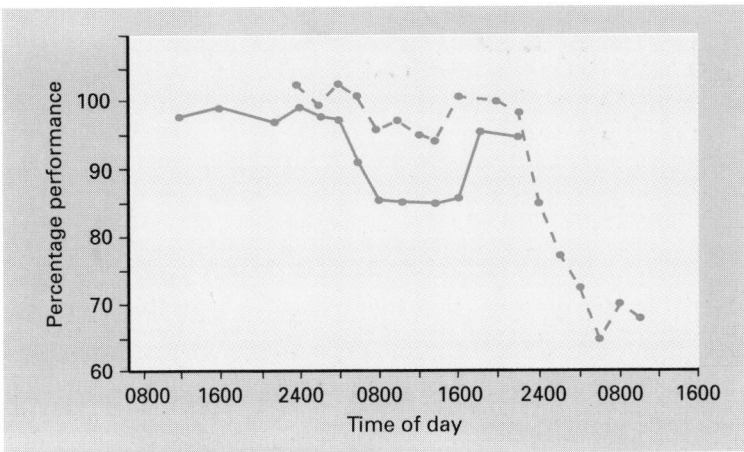

Performance at a vigilance task which lasted 34 hours. Two experiments are shown, one that began at noon (solid line) and one at midnight (dotted line).

Controlling the body clock

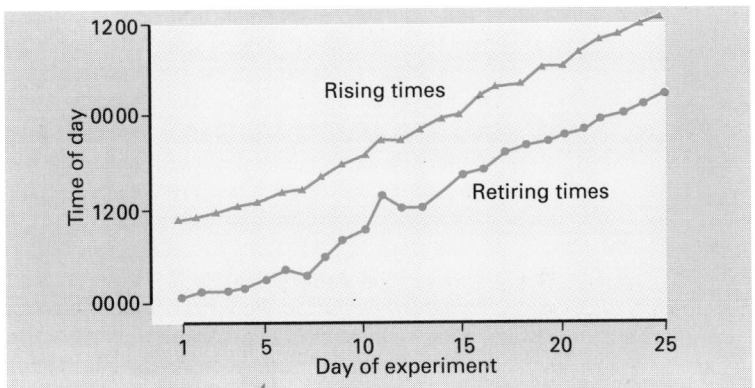

Times of retiring and rising on successive occasions in a person isolated from all external time cues, which shows synchronisation between the temperature and sleep/wake rhythms.

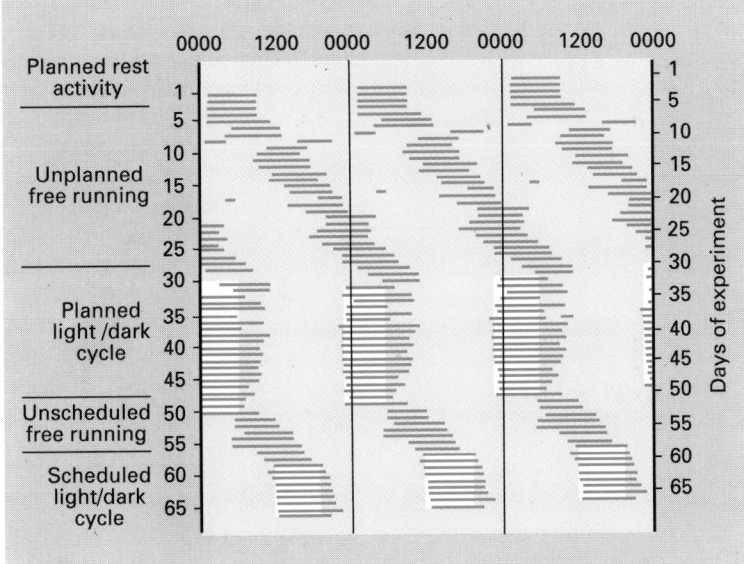

Times of sleep (black bars) of a single subject isolated from external time cues but free to choose times for meals and other activities. Successive days are plotted in triplicate from the top downwards. The experimental regimens were: days 1-5—normal routine of rest and activity; days 6-31—free running regimen; days 32-50—light/dark cycle (of an intensity similar to that used domestically) imposed by research workers (dark shown as light areas); days 51-58—free running regimen; days 59-end—light/dark cycle imposed by research workers.

Loss of sleep is associated with a decline in performance of many tasks, particularly those that are repetitive or require vigilance. Such decrements become more pronounced as the total time that has elapsed since the last sleep increases, and if the task is being performed at a time coincident with the trough in the temperature rhythm. The graph shows the levels of performance that were associated with two prolonged spells of vigilance, one starting at noon and the other at midnight. In both cases there was a general decline in performance as the experiment progressed, but when it ended at night and body temperature was low the deterioration was much more pronounced than when it ended during the day. Short sleeps or naps seem to reduce this deterioration, but the most effective length of a nap or the time to take it are important issues that remain to be resolved.

Free running experiments have also shown that without external time cues the body clock runs slow. Because it lasts about 25 hours it is called a circadian clock (from the Latin: circa=about, diem=a day). Such an inaccurate and potentially useless clock is adjusted to the solar day by environmental rhythms called synchronisers or Zeitgebers (from the German: Zeit=time, Geber=to give). The rhythmic pattern of dark and light (particularly of an intensity similar to that found outdoors and much brighter than that normally used domestically) is one means by which this can be achieved. In addition, humans in modern societies gain much information about time from their daily routine, affecting as it does social factors, activity, and meal times. For example, the observation that imposing a regular light/ dark cycle adjusted a person's sleep/wake cycle, with sleep times coinciding with the imposed darkness, does not mean that the light/dark the light/dark cycle probably acted in combination with rhythms of activity and meal times, and of other processes that are natural behavioural consequences of the light/dark cycle.

The complex interactions between the environment, the body clock, and the rhythms that it produces, enable rhythmic humans to integrate into a rhythmic environment. Not only are they "primed" during the day and partially "shut down" at night, but also their bodies can predict—and so prepare for—environmental changes. They can therefore prepare for sleep during the falling phase of adrenaline, alertness, and body temperature rhythms, and prepare for the next day as these rhythms continue beyond their minimum values.

Circadian rhythms
Jet lag and sleep problems

Symptoms of jet lag

- Daytime fatigue
- Inability to sleep at night
- Difficulty in concentrating
- Headache
- Loss of appetite
- Irregularities in bowel movement

The effects of possessing such a body clock can turn to our disadvantage if we change our pattern of sleep and activity, as when we cross several time zones. Under such circumstances a person experiences a general malaise, which includes headache, loss of appetite, irregularities of bowel movement, difficulty in concentrating, fatigue during the new day time, and yet an inability to sleep properly at night. These symptoms are known collectively as circadian dysrhythmia or "jet lag." The symptoms are worse after a flight to the east than after one to the west, and their severity is directly related to the number of time zones that have been crossed. The difficulties cannot be attributed either to the stress of the flight itself or to any "culture shock" because they do not arise after north/south flights and yet do arise in simulated time zone transitions in the laboratory (in which culture shock and the stress of flying are omitted).

The symptoms arise because of mismatching between the body clock (which initially continues to run on the time of the departure time zone) and the new environment with all its new time cues. As a result, after a flight to the east (for example, one that crosses six time zones) we will feel most tired and our ability to carry out many mental tasks will be lowest from 0600 to 1400 on the new time scale, and our new bed time will be at 1800 "body time"—a time normally associated with high alertness and mental performance. The loss of sleep will result in a decreased ability to function well. The quality of sleep will also change. Normally we have most slow wave sleep towards the beginning of a night's sleep. We also have most rapid eye movement (REM) sleep towards the end of sleep because it shows a circadian rhythm with a peak at about 1000 and a minimum at about 2200.

After a westward flight across six time zones, therefore, the amount of REM sleep will decline during the latter half of sleep, because the sleep period of 2400 to 0800 corresponds to 0600 to 1400 on body time. As a result, slow wave sleep is sometimes "squeezed out" of its normal position and distributed sporadically throughout more of the period of sleep than normal. This may contribute to the sense that sleep has been of poor quality. On subsequent nights the normal distribution of sleep stages begins to be restored.

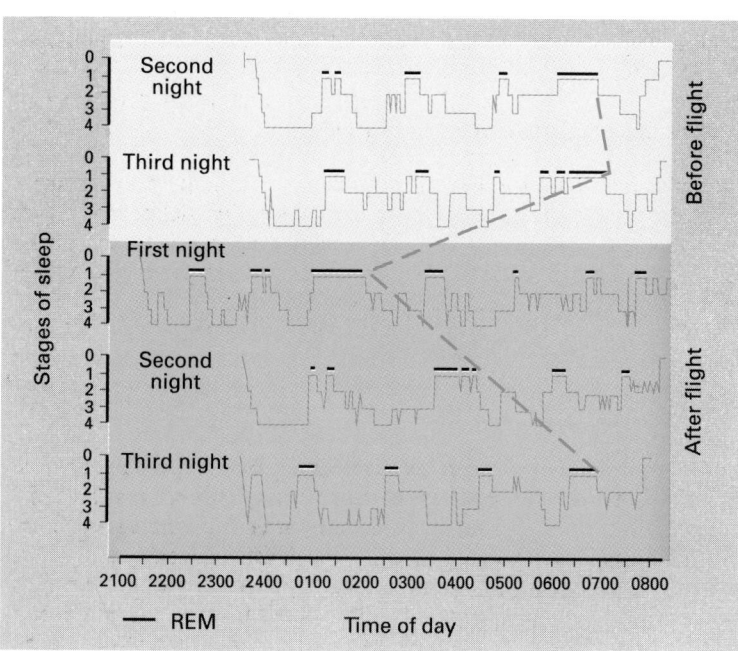

Distribution of sleep stages before and after a flight from east to west through six time zones. The dashed line indicates the shift in the time of maximum portions of REM sleep.

Combating jet lag

The symptoms of jet lag decline after a few days as the body clock and the rhythms that it drives synchronise with the new time zone under the influence of the new Zeitgebers. Attempts to deal with jet lag have concentrated on the sleep disturbance and associated fatigue. There are two main approaches: to minimise loss of sleep and to maximise the rate of adjustment of the body clock to the new time zone.

Good and bad local times for exposure to natural light in the first 2-3 days after a time zone transition

	Bad local times	Good local times
Time zones to the west		
4 hours	0100-0700*	1700-2300**
8 hours	2100-0300*	1300-1900**
12 hours	1700-2300*	0900-1500**
Time zones to the east		
4 hours	0100-0700**	0900-1500*
8 hours	0500-0800**	1300-1900*
12 hours	Same as 12 hours to the west	

*Will tend to advance the body clock.
**Will tend to delay the body clock.

Adjustment of the body clock

Adjustment of the body clock is generally accelerated by strengthening the Zeitgebers in the new time zone ("When in Rome..."). Adopting the new local hours for sleeping, for being awake and active, and for taking part in social functions, are the most important. Travellers should be encouraged to rest in a quiet, darkened room when it is bed time even if they do not feel tired, and to start the new day with gentle exercise even if they still feel sleepy. Naps are not recommended as they will tend to mislead the body about when it is night time. Exposure to natural daylight is beneficial but, particularly during the days immediately after the journey, its correct timing is important.

Meals

The correct timing of meals might be useful, because it stresses social Zeitgebers in the new time zone. It has been claimed that the appropriate type of food (a high protein/low carbohydrate breakfast and lunch; a high carbohydrate/low protein dinner; and drinks containing caffeine in the afternoon) will promote adjustment of the body clock, but this hypothesis has not yet been fully tested. It has recently become possible to buy pills that contain several compounds that are the "active constituents" of this "anti-jet-lag diet."

Drugs

Attempts have been made to overcome the poor sleep and increased fatigue. Hypnotic drugs can promote sleep, of course, but any effects that are carried over into the next period of activity are unwelcome. It is claimed that the third generation of hypnotic drugs that are currently coming on to the market do not have such effects. Short acting hypnotics have been tested extensively, and some benzodiazepines seem to be effective. Interestingly, it has recently been shown in rodents that receptors for benzodiazepines are present at the site of the body clock, and this might explain the observation that the drugs seem to adjust it. It would be an obvious advantage if a single substance could promote both sleep and the adjustment of the body clock.

Melatonin also reduces fatigue and improves sleep in long distance travellers. It has recently been shown that exogenous melatonin can adjust the clock in a time dependent way. Its effects are opposite to those of bright light so it should not be in the bloodstream when the patient is exposed to bright light. At present it is not generally available.

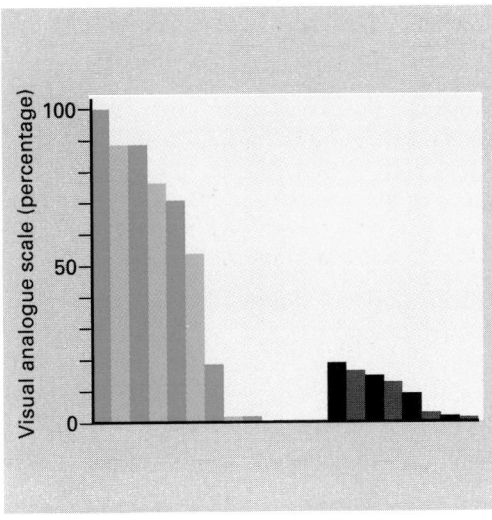

Visual analogue scores (0=insignificant, 100=very bad) showing severity of jet lag after a flight over eight time zones eastwards among eight subjects given melatonin (dark bars) and nine given placebo (blue bars).

Shift work

The fatigue and loss of sleep that accompany night work are obviously similar to those that follow time zone transitions, both in cause and effect. The problem is worse, however, in that they affect a larger section of the population and for extended periods. Chronic fatigue and sleep disturbances are often cited as reasons why some shift workers leave night work. The problem is exacerbated because the continual use of any drug to combat the effects is undesirable and rigid adherence to a routine that might promote adjustment of the body clock (or retain stable phasing of it in the case of those who work rapidly rotating shift systems) will make it much more inconvenient to shoulder or share domestic, family, and social responsibilities and pursue hobbies.

At present there is no clear solution to these conflicting interests but many patterns of shift work can be improved by careful consultation with the workforce and consideration of circadian influences. Recent studies have suggested that a short period of sleep in the middle of a night shift may mean that performance later on in the shift will be better maintained, as well as permitting the circadian rhythms to stabilise. This would make it easier for them to remain adapted to normal daily routines and would be advantageous to the worker, for example, during rest days.

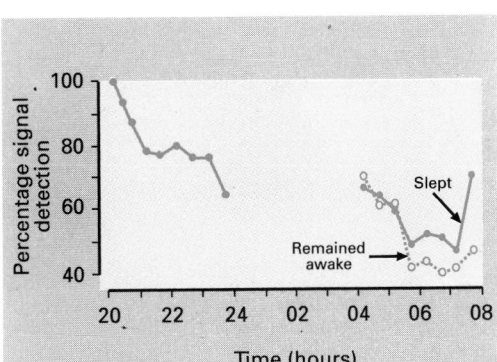

Effect of a four hour sleep on signal detection in a vigilance task. In both cases two four hour sessions were worked with a four hour break between them. During the break subjects were either allowed to sleep or required to stay awake.

The sources of the data presented in the graphs are: Froberg JE, *et al*, *Biol Psychol* 1975;2:175-88 for circadian rhythms of catecholamine excretion; Akerstedt T *et al*, *Sleep* 1981;4:159-69 for the circadian variation of experimentally displaced sleep; Czeisler CA *et al*, *Science* 1980;210:1264-7 for mean core temperature and sleep length; Morgan BB, Coates GD, eds. *Sustained performance and recovery during continuous operations* Norfolk: International Technical Report 74-2:1974, 21-38 for performance at a vigilance task; Waterhouse JM *et al*, *Your body clock*. Oxford: Oxford University Press: 1990, for times of retiring and rising; Czeisler CA *et al*, *Photochem Photobiol* 1981;34:239-47 for the light/dark activity cycle; Klein *et al*, *Aviation Space and Environmental Medicine* 1976;47:221-30 for distribution of sleep stages; Arendt *et al*, *BMJ* 1986;292:1170 for the visual analogue scores; and Colquhoun WP *et al*, eds. *Experimental studies on shiftwork*. Opladen: Westdeutscher Verlag: 1975, 20-8 for effect of a four hour sleep on signal detection in a vigilance task. The data are reproduced with permission.

SLEEPINESS AND PERFORMANCE

Eileen P Sloan, Colin M Shapiro

Epworth sleepiness scale

How likely are you to doze off or fall asleep in the following situations? Use the following scale to choose the most appropriate number for each situation:

0=would never doze   1=slight chance of dozing
2=moderate chance of dozing 3=high chance of dozing

Situation				
Sitting and reading	0	1	2	3
Watching TV	0	1	2	3
Sitting, inactive, in a public place	0	1	2	3
Passenger in a car for an hour without a break	0	1	2	3
Lying down to rest in the afternoon	0	1	2	3
Sitting and talking to someone	0	1	2	3
Sitting quietly after a lunch with no alcohol	0	1	2	3
In a car, while stopped for a few minutes in the traffic	0	1	2	3

A mean (SD) score of 17·5 (3·5) is found in patients with narcolepsy; 16 (4·4) in patients with severe obstructive sleep apnoea; and 5·9 (2·2) in normal controls. (John MW. *Sleep* 1991: **14** (6); 540-5.)

Categorisation for alertness and sleepiness by the maintenance of wakefulness test (MWT) and the multiple sleep latency test (MSLT).

	Frequency of sleep complaint	Social impact	Sleep latency on MSLT* (mins)	Alertness on MWT** (mins)
Mild	Intermittent	Minor	10-13	20-30
Moderate	Daily	Moderate	5-9	12-19
Severe	Daily	Severe	<5	<12

*MSLT=five naps throughout the day, each lasting 20 minutes. The patient is in a darkened room and is encouraged to try to fall asleep.
**MWT=four tests lasting 30 minutes during which time the patient is in a darkened room in a reclining position and is told to remain awake. For a lack of normal arousal to be considered the patient must fall asleep on at least two of the four tests.

Both commonsense and anecdotal evidence suggest that our abilities to concentrate, recall, and reason are related to the quality and quantity of our sleep. People often say that they feel lethargic and unable to function properly after a poor night's sleep. Subjective perception of the quality of sleep depends on many factors: sleep architecture, personality, mental state, and possibly also the precise point of the sleep cycle at which the person awakes. When a person has to perform particularly well the following day, the tendency is to "try and get a good night's sleep" to be properly prepared. We therefore associate a good night's sleep with good performance, and disturbed sleep and the subsequent sleepiness with impaired performance.

Despite the increase in knowledge about the mechanisms that control sleep and the aetiology of sleep disorders in the past few decades, research on the association between sleep and performance is limited, probably because sleepiness is difficult to quantify both subjectively and objectively. Two subjective scales are available (the Epworth sleepiness scale and the Stanford sleepiness scale), and laboratory tests such as the multiple sleep latency test (MSLT) give more objective assessments, and there is good correlation between them. Alertness is probably not the opposite of sleepiness, and is better measured by the maintenance of wakefulness test (MWT).

There is little evidence that poor sleep or sleep deprivation results in immediate physiological damage, but feelings of tiredness and fatigue are unpleasant and affect mood. The ability to do simple or monotonous tasks is impaired but the effect is diminished if the task is more difficult and requires more attention and effort, which indicates the critical role of attention and motivation in performance.

Certain aspects of complex tasks, however, are affected by sleep loss or deprivation, particularly the ability to think laterally. Some research workers have suggested that loss of sleep affects the willingness rather than the ability to perform. Incentives to perform may temporarily reduce the impact of sleepiness but are ineffective if sleeplessness is prolonged.

Shift work and performance

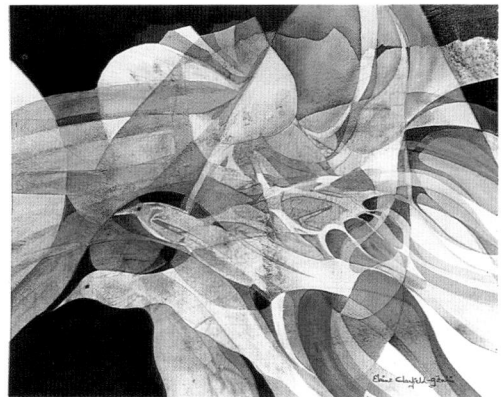

"Night Flight" by Elaine Clarfield-Citalis.

In a Danish study electroencéphalograms and electro-oculograms were monitored for a 24 hour period in machine operators who worked shifts during the night and the afternoon, and these showed a significant increase in power density and measures of sleepiness during the night shift. In addition, a fifth of the workers had one or more unintentional naps during the night shift. Sleepiness is a problem among shift workers; a recent study in Japan concluded that extending the night shift to include a nap for an hour or two could improve alertness and help to retain day-wake circadian patterns.

During recent years a number of serious industrial accidents have occurred throughout the world that may have been associated with sleepiness during night shifts. For example, the disaster at the Chernobyl nuclear plant occurred at 0135, and was apparently related to work patterns. The National Aeronautics and Space Administration (NASA) Challenger space shuttle disaster may have been related to errors of judgment made during the early hours of the morning by people who had had insufficient sleep while working at night during the days before the launch.

The role of sleepiness and fatigue in industrial accidents is still rarely considered. If errors of the magnitude of those mentioned can occur, it is likely that many minor accidents occur in ordinary industrial settings that cause injuries to workers and expense to employers. The number of errors in meter readings in a gas works peaks at night, and telephone operators connect calls more slowly at night. The number of sleep related motor accidents increases at night, particularly in the early hours, and this is matched by another peak at 1500-1600, emphasising the diurnal rhythm of alertness.

There are few short tests to measure the impact of sleep deprivation. In particular, cognitive ability is affected, and though many people will describe difficulty in selecting a key from their own bunch of keys when tired, it is difficult to translate this into a formal test.

The effects of shift work can be minimised in several ways (see box). A particular problem is getting off to sleep at unusual times of day.

Tips for combating shift related sleepiness

1 Nap before going to work at night
2 Arrange, if possible, to have shifts rotating clockwise—that is, morning, daytime, evening, night time
3 Have the night shift at the end of the shift schedule
4 Have a slow rotation of shifts if possible
5 Delay the sleep phase before going on to night shift—that is, go to bed progressively later each night
6 Improve your physical fitness as this seems to combat sleepiness during the night
7 Exposure to bright light in the evening and shielding from bright light in the morning, thereby altering your circadian phase, is helpful for some people
8 Do not drink alcohol before going to work, either during the day or at night, as this decreases performance and increases drowsiness
9 If you take medication consult your doctor about the best time of day to take it

---

Competence in performing repetitive tasks is decreased in sleepy workers

---

Sleepiness and memory

The number of reports about the effects of sleep loss and shift work on memory and performance is increasing, and many of them are of laboratory investigations which indicate that performance of various tasks deteriorates during the night. In particular, sleepy subjects show an increased number of delays in response and errors of omission. These lapses slow down such self paced tasks as mental arithmetic and logical reasoning, as well as affecting memory. Immediate recall is reduced, though recall of information acquired before the sleep deprivation is normal. Boring and repetitive tasks are likely to be most affected—for example, a house officer deprived of sleep may miss the arm of a patient when trying to put a needle into a vein but can focus and complete the task successfully. This example emphasises the effect of attention on performance.

Effect of drugs and alcohol

Some drugs and alcohol can cause sleepiness and deterioration in performance

---

Certain drugs and alcohol can cause increased drowsiness and deterioration in cognitive, psychomotor, and visuospatial performance. Stimulants used to treat narcolepsy (such as amphetamine or methylphenidate) tend to cause subjective underestimates of sleepiness. Objective measures, however, show that they increase the time taken to get to sleep, reduce the total time spent asleep and sleep efficiency, and increase the number of body movements. Methylphenidate increases physical endurance, reaction time, and the ability to carry out simple cognitive tasks, even after sleep deprivation.

The effects of antihistamines, antidepressant, and other psychotropic

Sleepiness and performance

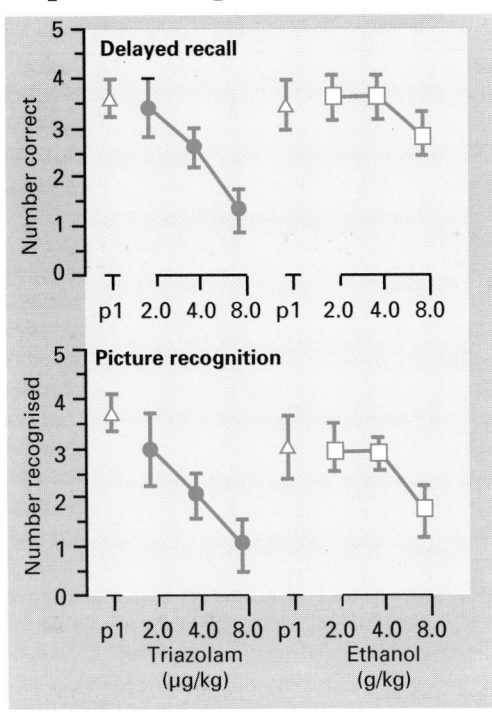

Dose related impairment produced by triazolam and ethanol on delayed number recall and picture recognition tasks.

drugs are described in the chapter on psychotropic drugs. Benzodiazepines have a dose dependent effect on psychomotor performance in healthy subjects, and most studies have confirmed that the longer acting drugs have more effect than the shorter acting ones. One feature that is poorly explained is the increase in fatigue that patients may feel after taking a hypnotic drug; this is probably the result of a combination of increased circadian sleepiness and lingering traces of the drug.

Alcohol causes a dose related increase in the amount and duration of subjective drowsiness as well as affecting performance, particularly if taken with hypnotics. In healthy volunteers it leads to impairment of motor coordination, attention, memory, problem solving, and reaction times. Central processing is more affected than peripheral motor functioning. The psychomotor and cognitive impairments caused by alcohol are related to dose and concentration in the blood, and can be detected when the subject is well below the legal limit of intoxication.

Some of these effects may be exacerbated by disruption of the sleep/wake cycle and by the normal circadian tendency to drowsiness at night, so the doctor must be aware of the effects of these drugs and alcohol when prescribing for patients on shift work. We usually favour a course of hypnotics for several weeks for patients with insomnia. Two exceptions are patients with jet lag and those whose sleep disruption is the result of shift work. Shift workers should also follow the instructions for sleep hygiene as far as possible (see chapter on practical management of insomnia), and in particular avoid alcohol.

Sleep deprivation in athletes

> ### Advice for athletes about sleep before an event
> - Encourage the athlete to attempt to sleep normally before an event
> - If changing time zone an allowance of time shift (1 day/hour shift) should be made
> - If hypnotics are to be used in adapting to the new time zone they should be tried out one month beforehand
> - If hypnotics are used on the night before the event they should be taken earlier rather than later
> - Sleepiness immediately before the event may be due to anxiety, not disinterest

Sleep deprivation does not cause as much reduction in athletic performance as might be expected but the regularity of lap time of middle distance runners is affected, which must affect the final performance of highly competitive athletes (see box).

SLEEP AND SLEEP PROBLEMS IN ELDERLY PEOPLE

Cameron G Swift, Colin M Shapiro

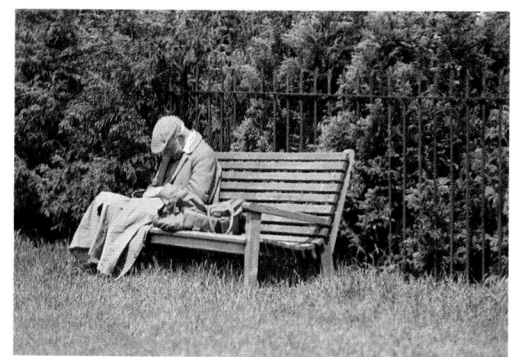

The reasons for special consideration of sleep and its problems among elderly people are:

● Increased dissatisfaction with the quality of sleep, complaints about insomnia, and use of hypnotic drugs, particularly among women
● Sleep architecture changes with increasing age
● Insomnia may be a marker of physical or psychological disorders, and of social or environmental problems
● The importance of the beneficial effects of healthy sleep, particularly on optimal central nervous system performance, during the day
● There is a need for a more circumspect and thoughtful approach to sleep problems in later life.

Prevalence of sleep problems and use of hypnotic drugs

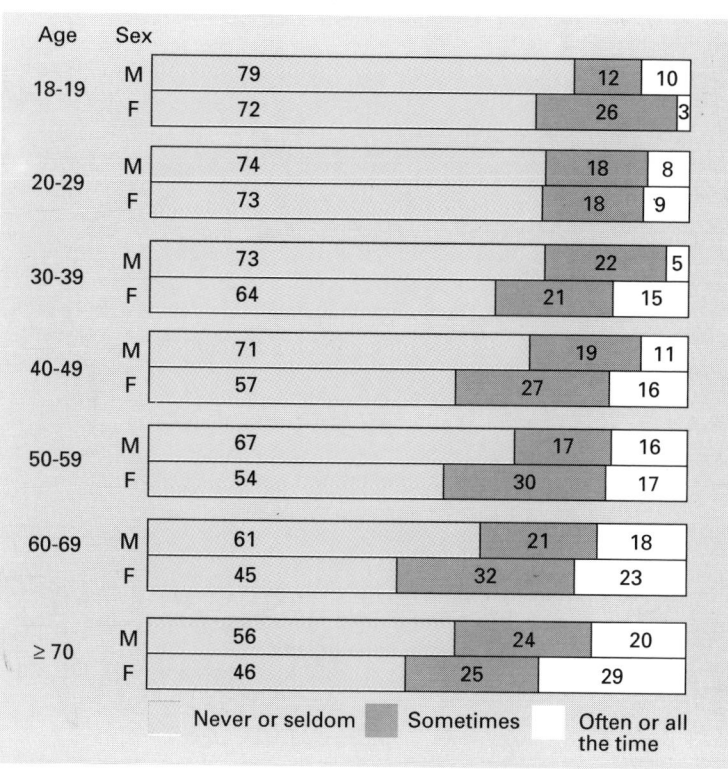

Percentages of people in different age groups who reported trouble with sleeping.

Surveys in Britain and the United States during the 1960s and 1970s showed a positive correlation between increasing age and subjective sleep problems. This was particularly pronounced among women, and their main complaints were of inadequate depth of sleep, frequent awakenings during the night, and not enough sleep. Getting off to sleep was not a common problem among older people.

Not surprisingly, evidence from many large studies showed that there was a corresponding increase in the prescription and use of hypnotic drugs with age; the mean figure in the community was between 10% and 15% among elderly people and higher among those over 75, women, and those in hospital and residential and nursing homes. The drugs were being taken regularly, for long periods, irrespective of any precipitating cause of the insomnia, and without any clinical review of need. The use of hypnotics probably peaked between 1960 and 1980 before the potential of benzodiazepines to cause dependence had been realised. Nevertheless people taking hypnotic drugs long term often express satisfaction with the results despite the fact that many of these drugs become less effective with time.

Sleep and sleep problems in elderly people

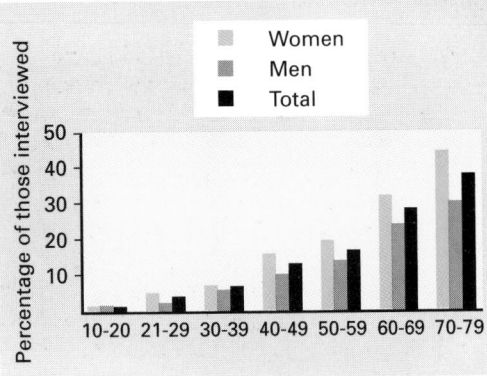

Consumption of sleeping drugs according to age.

Risks of treatment

The risks of treatment with hypnotic drugs among older people include accentuated acute sedation (as a result of enhanced central nervous system sensitivity, or changes in pharmacokinetics, or both) and unwanted residual sedation, particularly during the initial stages of treatment. With regular doses there may be appreciable accumulation of the parent drug or its metabolite, which can impair daytime performance, cognition, motor activity, and postural stability in susceptible people. Dependence, rebound insomnia, and other signs of withdrawal are common, particularly with rapidly cleared compounds. All these risks have to be set against the rather ill defined and possibly ephemeral benefits.

Changes in sleep architecture and physiology

Studies of older people in the sleep laboratory have shown that they have definite changes in electroencephalographic characteristics, in the sleep cycle, and in the composition of sleep. These include:

> Sleep patterns may change with age. There is more variability in sleep patterns in the old and young

- Decreased amplitude in the size of slow waves (the restorative component of sleep)
- Abnormal or "degraded" spindles during stage 2 sleep (the characteristic feature of this stage)
- Decreased number of eye movements during rapid eye movement (REM) sleep, suggesting that it is less intense
- Increased time spent in bed with a decrease in total time spent asleep, showing a reduction in sleep efficiency
- Increased number and duration of awakenings (more pronounced in men) and a reduced arousal threshold for noise (more pronounced in women)
- Appreciable reduction in the total amount of slow wave sleep (in addition to the decreased amplitude)
- Reductions in both the total duration of REM sleep, and the time from the onset of sleep to REM sleep
- Increased number of shifts from one stage of sleep to another
- Increased frequency of daytime napping, more pronounced among men, and the very old (25% of 70 year old, compared with 45% of 80 year old, men).

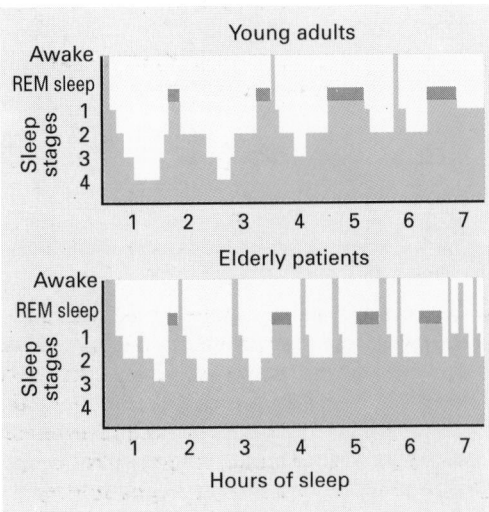

Typical hypnograms for young adults and elderly people.

These findings are broadly consistent with reported subjective complaints of sleep disturbance. In addition, there is some evidence of a reduction in amplitude and for desynchronisation of circadian rhythms (for example, secretion of melatonin). During each decade after the age of 60 there is a further advance of one hour in sleep phase.

All these observations are, however, extreme generalisations and the variability among individual people is if anything greater among older people than among younger ones. The fact that such changes do occur not only helps us to understand sleep patterns better, but may also help to identify objectives to aim for in the treatment of sleep disturbances in older people.

Insomnia

> If an elderly person complains of insomnia a diagnostic response is necessary

It is important to make a diagnostic response to a complaint of insomnia in an elderly person, partly because it may lead to the recognition of an underlying physical or mental problem, and partly because it may pre-empt the blanket prescription of hypnotic drugs without good reason.

The following possibilities should be considered:

Any physical illness that causes discomfort may naturally disrupt sleep, and older people are often reluctant to voice such complaints spontaneously. Obvious examples are: nocturnal dyspnoea caused by left ventricular failure; tachyarrhythmias that cause angina or palpitations; gastro-oesophageal reflux; peptic ulcer; constipation; exacerbations of chronic obstructive airways disease; skeletal pain caused by osteoarthritis, osteoporosis, metastatic deposits, or Paget's disease; and cutaneous pruritis.

Some age related complaints are particularly associated with insomnia, such as bladder detrusor instability and prostatism, both of which may cause nocturia. Nocturnal myoclonus, "restless legs syndrome," and night cramps are positively related to age, as is "sleep apnoea." The number of apnoeic events tends to be much lower than found among young people with sleep apnoea, however, and there is controversy about the clinical importance of the syndrome in older people. A degree of respiratory irregularity during sleep may be compatible with aging, and the clinical usefulness of treating mild apnoea is questionable. Some cognitive changes may occur during sleep apnoea and it has been speculated that these may be one of the causative factors in dementia. Hypnotic drugs may exacerbate respiratory problems during sleep.

Psychiatric disorders, in particular depression and dementias, commonly present with insomnia in old age. The threshold for the diagnosis and treatment of depression may not be sufficiently low; in one survey it was found that only a fifth of elderly depressed patients were receiving appropriate drugs, the rest having been given a hypnotic. Dementia was associated with increased wakefulness during the night, and with greater reductions in slow wave and REM sleep than found in age matched subjects who were not demented. In the late stages of dementia there is greater circadian breakdown, though 8% of demented patients seem to maintain a sleep pattern appropriate for their age.

Iatrogenic causes of insomnia include theophyllines, sympathomimetics, diuretics, lipophilic β blockers, and sedatives and hypnotics that cause rebound withdrawal. Caffeine, both in drinks and in over the counter drugs, and high alcohol concentrations have also been implicated.

It is difficult to establish a precise relation between insomnia and social and environmental factors, but isolation, inadequate heating, being in an institution, bereavement, and financial hardship all impair sleep.

Various age related behavioural factors may play a part, including reduced physical activity and reduced exposure to daylight.

Causes of nocturnal agitation

New onset
- Environmental change
- Delirium
- Bereavement

Recurrent
Disease related
- Dementia
- Depression
- Late life mania
- Late life panic disorder
- Anxiety disorder
- Sleep apnoea
- Nocturnal enuresis
- Chronic pain syndromes

Precipitating factors
- Environmental lighting
- Physical restraint
- Drugs—for example, phenothiazines
- Withdrawal of any psychoactive drugs
- Sensory deprivation—physical or environmental
- Altered circadian rhythm
- Frequent awakenings
- Night hunger—meals too early
- Social fear of the dark
- "Burnout" of staff or carer

Sleep and daytime performance

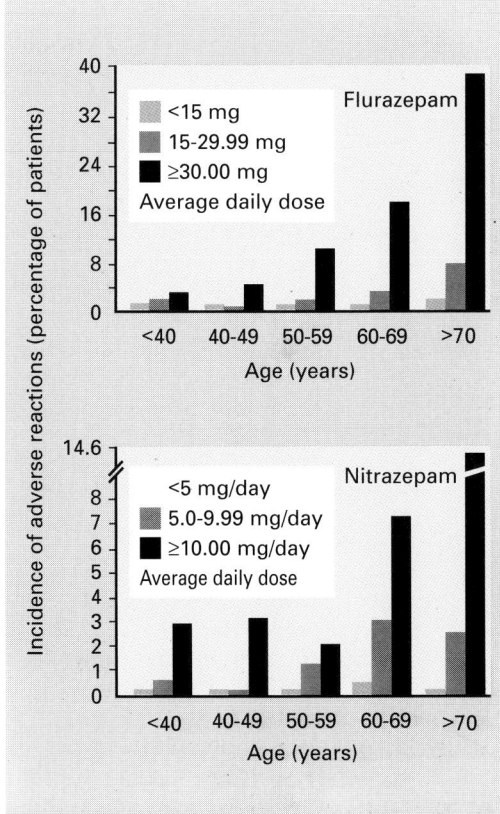

Incidence of unwanted depression of the central nervous system by flurazepam and nitrazepam according to mean daily dose and age.

The evidence that correction of sleep deficiency improves daytime alertness is good, but there is little specifically about older people. Central nervous system performance during the day may be the key to autonomy and wellbeing in an older person. There is an increased number of road traffic accidents among elderly people, which may be related to lessened alertness. If alleviation of acute or chronic insomnia could be shown objectively to improve performance among elderly people, therefore, it would be an appropriate end point for treatment.

Much has been written about impairment of daytime performance in older people by hypnotic drugs, and the Boston collaborative drug surveillance programme in the 1970s emphasised that this effect was dose related. Benzodiazepines are the most likely to cause immediate oversedation and unwanted residual sedation because of the increase in their pharmacodynamic "sensitivity" with age. The reduction in the rate of clearance is probably less important, but may compound the accentuated responsiveness. It is therefore essential—at least to begin with—to use reduced doses in older people irrespective of the plasma half lives of the drugs being used. The information about the non-benzodiazepine hypnotics is less comprehensive, but the response to compounds in this category that are cleared rapidly (such as chlormethiazole) may be less age related, and therefore more predictable from pharmacokinetic data.

We are therefore justified in seeking better ways of improving the quality of sleep in elderly people. The evidence that hypnotics have a part to play in improving daytime performance is sparse.

Sleep and sleep problems in elderly people
Dealing with sleep problems

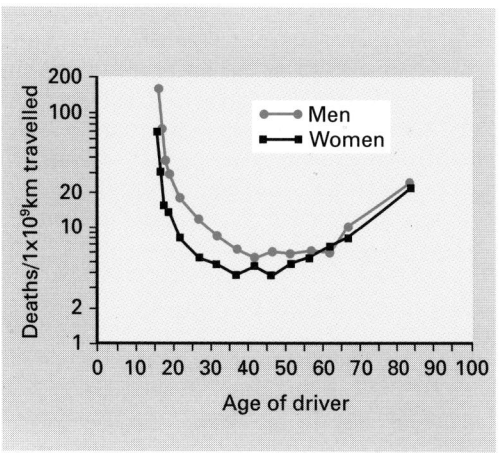

Sleep related accidents according to age.

As the disadvantages and hazards of the hitherto rather casual prescribing of hypnotic drugs become more widely recognised, a more considered response to sleep problems should gain ground (though this does not exclude the careful use of hypnotics). Experience so far, however, suggests that in the absence of a structured and rigorous approach to assessment such guidelines are unlikely to be followed.

We suggest the following proposals:

- Allow time to make at least one systematic diagnostic assessment for underlying causes of sleep problems, and try to treat them first before having recourse to hypnotics
- Consider a non-pharmacological approach to "primary" sleep disorders. This may include counselling to allay anxiety about incorrect or inappropriate expectations about sleep (such as the statutory "seven or eight hours a night"). Simple behavioural and cognitive approaches may help, and physical activity and exposure to daylight should be encouraged. These may well rescue people from long term dependence on hypnotics
- Use hypnotic drugs judiciously as third line or adjunctive treatment, and in accordance with defined guidelines.

Conclusion

Guidelines for prescribing hypnotics for elderly patients

1 Limit to times of particular stress
2 Prescribe a specific dose (not "one or two")
3 Use small initial doses
4 Advise "if required" rather than habitual use but if possible give a set course of treatment—for example, 3-4 weeks
5 Review the response with special reference to side effects
6 Aim to discontinue after a short course

Many elderly people have longstanding sleep problems. Increasing awareness of these problems may be beneficial, particularly as increased sleep improves daytime alertness. Techniques for doing this require further study.

The sources of data presented in the figures are: Karacan *et al*, *Soc Sci Med* 1976;**10**:239-44 for percentage in different age groups that have trouble with sleeping; Spiegel R, Azcona A, *Sleep and its disorders*. In: Pathy MSJ, ed. Principles and practice of geriatric medicine. Chichester, John Wiley, 1985 for age and consumption of sleeping drugs; and Greenblatt et al, *Clin Pharmacol Ther* 1977;**21**:355-61 for incidence of unwanted depression of the central nervous system. The photograph is reproduced with permission of Alan Gale.

SLEEP DISORDERS IN CHILDREN

Tony Jaffa, Stephen Scott, Jean Harris Hendriks, Colin M Shapiro

Development of normal sleep

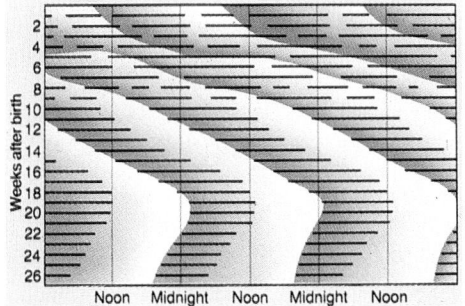

Initially an infant has a broken sleep regimen. After the first 12 weeks of life this usually consolidates into a regular sleep pattern. Solid lines indicate episodes of sleep.

Sleep is influenced by many factors, including age. Newborn babies sleep for about 16 hours a day with brief alternating periods of sleep and wakefulness, the electroencephalographic trace going directly from the alert pattern to rapid eye movement (REM) activity, missing out sleep stages 1-4. As babies become older they sleep for longer periods, though overall for fewer hours, and the sleep becomes concentrated into the night. By 3 months of age about 70% of babies sleep through until morning, though at 1 year 10% are still waking their parents each night. Sleep studies have shown that waking during the night is a fairly usual pattern, but what is more variable is whether the infant goes back to sleep or becomes more alert and calls out. By the age of 1 year the sleep electroencephalogram resembles that of an adult.

Sudden infant death syndrome

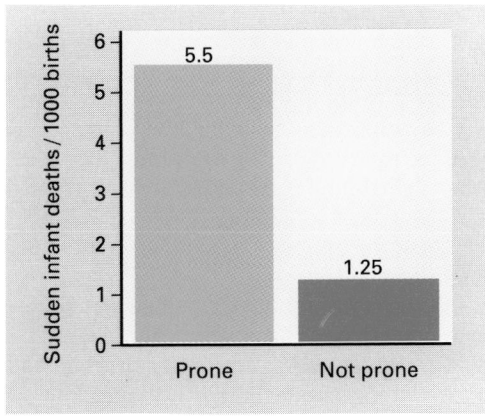

Effect of sleeping position on death rate from sudden infant death syndrome: results of a large prospective study in Tasmania.

Many physiological changes occur during sleep. These include variations in the regulation of breathing, circulation, and other autonomic functions. For example, thermoregulation is suspended during REM sleep, and cerebral blood flow increases dramatically. How any of these is precisely related to the sudden infant death syndrome is so far not known, though there are many theories. The deaths usually occur during sleep; over four fifths occur before the age of 6 months, and the rate is double between January and March compared with June to August. Retrospective studies both in the United Kingdom and abroad have shown significantly fewer deaths among babies who did not sleep prone. The effect of a campaign during which parents were told to place their babies on their backs or sides to sleep led to a remarkable reduction in the number of deaths in Avon, England. Late in 1991 this became a national policy in England and Wales, formally sponsored by the Department of Health, and results so far suggest a reduction nationally of about a half compared with 1988.

Sleep and growth

Adolescents really do need more sleep

Sleep is also a time of growth, which is facilitated by the establishment of early circadian rhythms. In young children who have been severely abused there is inhibition of nocturnal release of growth hormone, and psychosocial dwarfism may be the consequence. During the growth spurt in adolescence the steady decline in hours slept each night compared with childhood is temporarily reversed, often giving rise to misplaced complaints of lazy adolescents who do in fact require more sleep.

Sleep disorders in children
Patterns of sleep disturbance

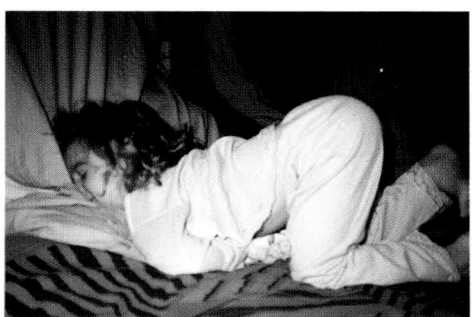

Characteristic sleeping position of a child with sleep apnoea.

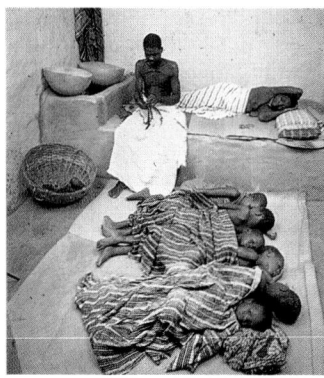

Living conditions may influence sleep.

Sleep disturbance can be broadly categorised into excessive sleep and inadequate or interrupted sleep.

Excessive sleep

Daytime drowsiness is most commonly the result of sleep deprivation, but it may also be caused by a number of rare syndromes that usually present from late childhood onwards.

Narcolepsy—This is characterised by a sudden irresistible desire to go to sleep that lasts for minutes to hours at a time. It is associated with cataplexy (the sudden loss of tone in one or more muscle groups) and with vivid auditory or visual hallucinations when falling asleep. These can be extremely disturbing, and a child who complains of odd experiences at night should not be dismissed as merely dreaming.

Klein-Levin syndrome—This affects adolescent boys. Periods of pronounced hypersomnia and overeating alternate with periods of normality. There may be dramatic changes in libido.

Sleep apnoea—Excessive tonsillar and adenoidal tissue may cause intermittent obstruction of the airway, which leads to sleep apnoea, daytime drowsiness, and even intellectual impairment. Children characteristically sleep on their elbows and knees with their buttocks in the air and neck hyperextended. Management is surgical, after which a growth spurt may be noted.

Inadequate or interrupted sleep

Nightmares occur during REM sleep. The child wakes in an anxious state with a tachycardia and tachypnoea and can usually remember at least some of the content of the dream. This may be related to specific traumatic experiences or to frightening films or television programmes. Nightmares are common, but unless they are frequent and persistent reassurance and comfort are all that is required.

Night terrors occur in about 3% of children, more commonly in boys, and tend to run in families. They occur in sleep stages 3 and 4—that is, in deep sleep. A child who experiences a night terror seems terrified, stares into space, and possibly mutters indistinctly. The child is not awake and if left alone will calm down and return to a resting sleep state. Though parents find a night terror disturbing, the child wakes in the morning with no memory of it. Night terrors increase at times of stress, but in isolation are not indicative of emotional disturbance; most children grow out of them.

Sleepwalking and sleeptalking, like night terrors, occur during sleep stages 3 and 4, are not remembered in the morning, and are not indicative of emotional disturbance. Parents of a habitual sleepwalker are well advised to secure doors and windows to reduce the risk of injury.

Problems of settling and remaining asleep

Much commoner than the specific conditions described above are general difficulties in settling and remaining asleep. The problem may be in settling, with long and increasingly acrimonious arguments about going to bed, after which children may repeatedly come out of their bedrooms. The problem may be later, when they wake up in the night and complain that they are afraid, or in pain, and it takes considerable reassurance before they go back to bed or get into bed with the parents. There are many contributory causes:

Physical and environmental factors must be considered. Children may be woken by somatic symptoms such as abdominal pain, the cough or breathlessness of asthma, or the irritation of eczema. Wetting the bed or worry that they are going to may cause considerable loss of sleep for enuretic children. There is much temporal variation in how much children sleep, and those at the extreme who wake frequently as babies tend to continue to sleep less than other children as they grow older. Sleep disturbance is relatively common among those with appreciable developmental delay and mental handicap.

Unfavourable living conditions associated with social deprivation such as a cold, damp bedroom, or sharing the room or bed with noisy siblings, will exacerbate if not cause sleep disturbances.

Sleep disorders in children

Psychological factors often maintain sleep problems whatever their original cause. Children may have got into the habit of waking up at night and have been encouraged by the parental response (see below). They may be anxious not to be separted from a parent, fearing that the parent will be injured, leave, or die during the night. This anxiety will be more common among children who have witnessed marital violence, undergone a long separation, or experienced life threatening illness or death of a loved one. Those children who wake at night to find that they are being sexually abused will have particular fears of falling asleep.

Psychiatric disorders—Occasionally among older chidren and adolescents sleep disturbance may be related to a specific psychiatric disorder. Generally poor sleep as well as early morning waking may be the result of a depressive illness. Misuse of drugs such as amphetamines will lead to overarousal and distorted sleep patterns. The checking associated with a severe obsessive-compulsive disorder may last until the early hours of the morning.

Parents' response—This is of prime importance. Firstly, they may fail to make going to bed an agreeable experience. The importance of a routine should not be overlooked—for example, a fixed time, regular sequence of events, calming activities such as a bath and a story, and the security of having a light on at night. Secondly, giving in for a few minutes after a prolonged battle about going to bed inadvertently rewards the child, and is enough to reinforce the behaviour pattern for long periods. Thirdly, parents may unwittingly encourage sleep problems by rewarding wakefulness and calling out with long chats, stories, cuddles, and affection. Sometimes, however, there is an underlying problem in the relationship, with one parent emotionally overinvolved with the child—for example, they may want the child in bed with them to relieve their own loneliness or anxiety, finding separation unbearable as the child is especially precious to them. In this case there will be a general failure to promote the child's independence and separate identity. An absent or distant relationship with the partner may exacerbate this.

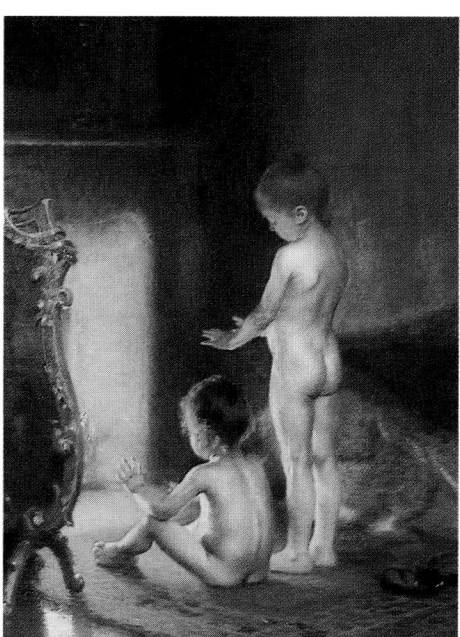

Comforting routines before bedtime help sleep. ("After the bath" by Paul Peel (1890)).

History and examination

Example of a sleep diary

Day	Monday
Time woke in morning	0600
Sleeps during the day	1110-1150, 1430-1600
Bedtime	1900
What happened at bedtime?	Cried for 10 minutes and came into lounge, sat quietly and fell asleep at 2045. Carried to bed
Contacts during the night	0130 Climbed into our bed and slept quietly until morning

A carefully and sensitively taken history will identify relevant factors. A sleep diary is a particularly useful way of obtaining information about the problem behaviour and its maintenance. Details of the child's sleeping and waking, and the parents' responses, are recorded for one or two weeks. The child's general development and emotional wellbeing should be evaluated, including social and educational functioning.

Assessment of the family should include their current predicament and concerns, including emotional issues, financial difficulties, and unemployment. Depression or anxiety in the parents, or discord in their relationship, are relevant because they are likely to be picked up by the child whose sleep disturbance may in turn perpetuate them. Separations, whether because of death, illness, divorce, or other reasons, are likely to increase the child's anxiety. Physical examination should include inspection of the throat for tonsillar enlargement and of the chest for signs of asthma, and measurement of height and weight.

Management

Devising a behaviour modification programme

- Identify the problem
- Specify desirable and undesirable behaviours
- Plan responses to unwanted behaviour
- Plan rewards for desired behaviour
- Plan details of implementation
- Implement
- Review and, if necessary, modify

A transient, isolated, mild problem may resolve with reassurance. Otherwise behaviour modification may be helpful.

The introduction of a regular bedtime routine may signal a new regimen, and a new determination on the part of the parents, which after some initial testing out by the child is often accepted surprisingly readily. The parents should be helped to stop rewarding the child with attention or drinks for repeatedly leaving the bedroom or calling out. With encouragement most parents find that they can give enough comfort to reassure the child and themselves, but not so much as to encourage repetition of the problem behaviour. Greater rewards in the form of praise and treats (not late nights) can be given when the child sleeps through the night, or at least does not call out. A reward system can be formalised by using a "star chart" on which

Sleep disorders in children

Behaviour modification

According to the theory of "operant conditioning," a response to a situation changes according to its consequences for the person concerned.

Example of how operant conditioning can maintain sleep problems

Take the situation of the child who is put to bed, and 10 minutes later gets up and joins the parents. The likelihood of the child's behaviour being repeated will depend on what happens next. A consequence which is experienced by the child as desirable (such as increased parental attention) will encourage repetition. A consequence which is not experienced as desirable (such as being promptly returned to the bedroom) will not have this effect. The parents may therefore modify the child's behaviour by avoiding rewarding behaviour that they find undesirable, and instead rewarding that which is wanted. In this case the parents should not only avoid rewards for getting up at night, but they should also institute rewards for staying in bed until morning. Inevitably, this is an extreme oversimplification of a much more complicated picture. It is, however, one which often permits effective action.

stars are earned for specified behaviour such as going to bed on time, staying in bed, and not calling out. Children should not be required to do things that are beyond their control, such as going to sleep at a particular time.

Studies have shown that these programmes are extremely effective if implemented fully and conscientiously, but many parents find them difficult to put into practice. Time should therefore be spent in planning, discussing possible difficulties, and devising strategies to overcome them. Some may find it easier to change their own and the child's behaviour in small steps, progressively decreasing the time before a child who gets up is put back to bed, or the number of stories read, and so on. The initial "testing out" period is particularly strenuous for parents. They need to understand that the child is trying to re-establish the old routine, so if they waver it will increase the child's attempts to return to the old pattern.

If behavioural management proves unsuccessful, or the sleep disorder is part of a wider problem, an alternative approach may be indicated. This is likely to require the participation of child mental health services and may include psychological assessment and treatment of one form or another with the child and perhaps the parents as well. Drugs to induce sleep are likely to be of only temporary benefit and should seldom be used in children

PYSCHIATRIC ASPECTS OF SLEEP DISORDERS AND SLEEP PATTERNS IN PSYCHIATRIC CONDITIONS

A H Crisp, Colin M Shapiro

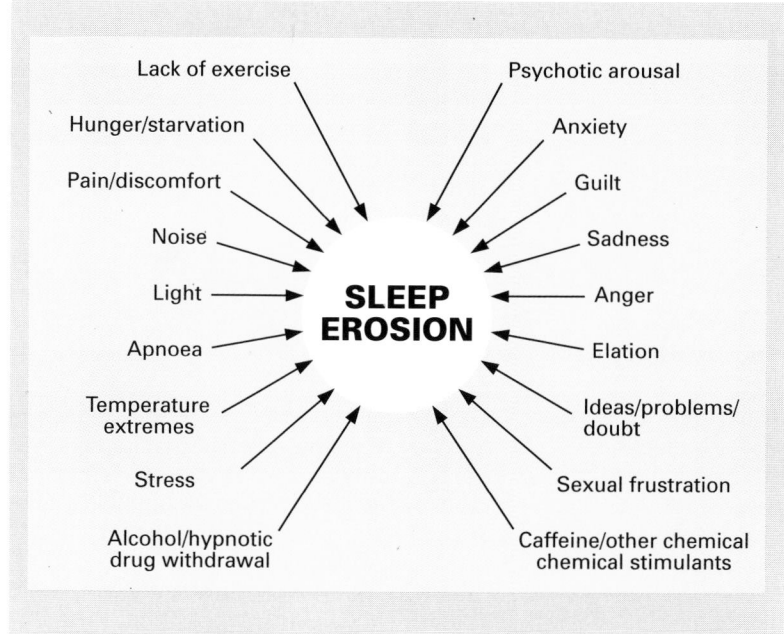

Some factors that can erode sleep.

There are many facets of sleep disorders which interact with psychiatric processes and almost all psychiatric illnesses have as a feature an alteration in sleep pattern. In this chapter we discuss the psychiatric issues in various sleep disorders and then specifically mention sleep changes in certain psychiatric conditions.

Hypersomnias

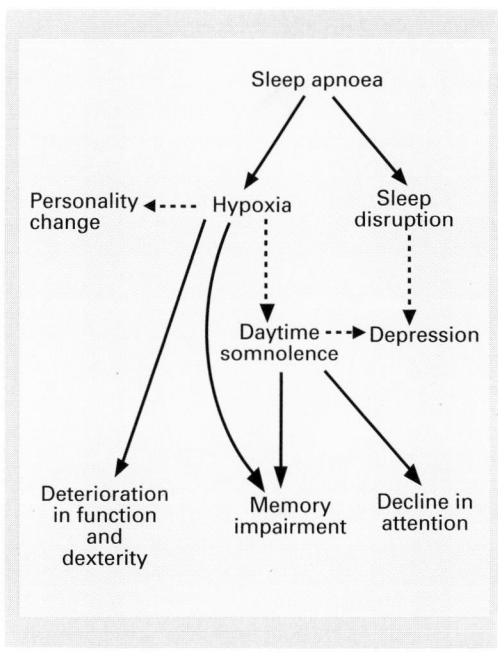

Neuropsychiatric changes in sleep apnoea.

Cognitive deficits are often identified in patients with narcolepsy and sleep apnoea. This may be as a consequence of excessive sleepiness leading to poor attention and vigilance. However, the sleep disruptive aspects of these conditions, particularly the disruption of REM sleep, may be a further factor in influencing learning processes.

The repeated hypoxic episodes at night in those with sleep apnoea may be partially responsible for the memory impairment, and especially significant in the decline in executive functions and dexterity seen in these patients.

Many patients with excessive daytime sleepiness have concomittant depression. The personality change that is often observed but little studied in these patients may have very different causes. The psychostimulant drugs used in narcolepsy often produce an irritability and a sense of being "driven." Many are frustrated about not being able to be as active as previously; their decline in intellectual capacity, even if only as a consequence of decreased attention; and the concern that in part this is a genetic disorder.

Psychiatric aspects of sleep

In patients with sleep apnoea there is the possibility of hypoxic brain damage which may underpin personality changes. The reversal of symptoms—for example, of sleepiness—with CPAP is often the end point of treatment, but family and marital problems often persist, possibly as a consequence of personality change. Many of these patients, despite being aware of the increased risk of cerebrovascular accidents, myocardial infarction, and nocturnal death associated with sleep apnoea have an inordinate difficulty in losing weight—seemingly more so than patients with similar degrees of obesity trying to lose weight. Sleep disruption itself and consequent daytime fatigue may account for these personality effects.

Occasionally narcolepsy is misdiagnosed as schizophrenia. In one study it was estimated that seven per cent of "schizophrenic patients" in a long stay institution were misdiagnosed patients with narcolepsy, in whom phenothiazine treatment for what were originally hypnagogic hallucinations had induced more generalised hallucinations, increased sleepiness, and an apparent deficit state.

Parasomnias, circadian rhythm and other sleep disorders

The most common triggers for parasomnias in adults are sleep deprivation, alcohol consumption, and stress. Psychotropic drugs, particularly lithium and neuroleptics, occasionally trigger parasomnias and may lead to bizarre behaviour in patients who have recently started taking these drugs for a psychotic illness

In adults the frequency of parasomnias is often related to psychic stress and psychopathology. There are no trials showing that psychotherapy is effective in treating these disorders, but many psychiatrists working in the specialty of sleep disorders evaluate such patients for the possibility of brief or intermediate psychotherapy. There is evidence that different parasomnias show distinct psychoneurotic characteristics (that is, adult sleepwalkers and patients with night terrors score differently on psychometric scales). In the case of patients with sleep eating, there is the suspicion of greater psychopathology with features of abuse, drug dependence, and eating disorders more commonly recorded than in other parasomnias, but data in this area are patchy.

Circadian rhythms are often altered in patients with psychiatric illness. Bright light therapy in the evening can phase delay rhythms and may be a solution to early morning awakenings in elderly and depressed patients with terminal insomnia

Patients with circadian abnormalities are often seen as eccentric, difficult, and non-compliant with treatment programmes. Occasionally frank psychosis is linked with circadian disturbances. It is not possible at present to determine to what extent the psychopathology observed is a consequence of longstanding conflicts with aberrant circadian patterns or timekeeping, whether some underlying biological process is influencing both behavioural and body clock problems, or if some other interaction is occurring.

Other disorders with a focus on sleep or arousal patterns—for example, the chronic fatigue syndrome and seasonal affective disorder—have clear sleep changes which in some cases are relatively specific, but these are often part of the psychiatric condition.

Psychiatric conditions with sleep changes

Patients with insomnia or hypersomnolence extending two months beyond treatment of a primary psychiatric condition should have further assessment and investigation of their sleep disruption

Depression

Characteristic changes in sleep architecture occur in patients with depression. These include a shortening of REM onset latency (the time from sleep onset to REM sleep); a reversal of the usual pattern so that more slow wave sleep occurs in the second sleep cycle, rather than the first; and more disruption of sleep through the night. Several studies have shown that if there is no improvement in sleep architecture while a patient is being treated with anti-depressants the patient is more likely to relapse into a depressed state when the anti-depressants are stopped.

Most forms of treatment of depression induce a suppression of REM sleep. This includes all categories of anti-depressants and electroconvulsive therapy. Sleep deprivation itself has been shown to have beneficial effects in treating depression, particularly in patients with a more pronounced diurnal variation in mood, and is occasionally used in patients who, for some reason, eschew drug treatments or electroconvulsive therapy. In one large epidemiological study the conclusion that insomnia and hypersomnia may trigger depression and not simply be manifestations of depression has led to an increasing awareness, particularly with regard to patients with previous depression, that early vigorous treatment of insomnia is merited.

In pregnancy the disruption of sleep associated with a night time delivery is more likely to result in postnatal blues. This implies that in patients with a history of postpartum psychosis a daytime delivery should be ensured to reduce the risk of repeated postpartum psychosis.

The sensitivity and specificity of sleep changes in depression are sufficiently robust, particularly in older patients and in the more severe forms of depression, to be occasionally useful diagnostically. Not all features of depression will resolve contemporaneously and loss of libido or sleep disturbance may take much longer than the improvement of mood to resolve. The doctor must therefore ensure that anti-depressant treatment should extend beyond initial or partial symptomatic relief.

> At least 90% of patients with depression have some sleep abnormality. In fact 20% of these have hypersomnolence rather than insomnia. The corresponding figure for patients with seasonal affective disorder is over 60% with hypersomnolence

Panic disorder

About 5-10% of patients with panic disorder have panic attacks exclusively arising from sleep and many more have panic attacks both during the night and during the day. Available evidence suggests that nocturnal panic attacks often arise at the time of transition between stage 2 and stage 3 or 4 sleep. Differential diagnosis includes night terrors, nocturnal asthmatic attacks if respiratory symptoms are prominent (some nocturnal asthmatic attacks appear to be triggered by REM sleep), and nightmares. It has been suggested that nocturnal panic attacks may be a consequence of autonomic dysregulation during sleep, whereas daytime panic attacks may be more psychogenic in origin. In some, nocturnal panic attacks may expand to include daytime attacks and treatment for these two aetiologically distinct forms of panic may need to be different.

> Patients with panic attacks arising during sleep may do better with biological rather than psychological treatment approaches

Schizophrenia

There are few studies in schizophrenic patients not taking drugs on which to base any description of sleep changes. In general, the separation of sleepiness and tiredness or fatigue is poorly tackled by doctors and by psychometric tests, and in many patients with schizophrenia the process of withdrawal and apathy combined with leading questions about sleep change leads to reported changes in sleep which may be overstated. The limited research indicates that there is a decline in sleep efficiency—that is, more disrupted sleep and a decline in REM latency—which is similar to that seen in patients with depression.

> Sleep efficiency is reduced in schizophrenic patients

MEDICAL PROBLEMS DURING SLEEP

P M A Calverley, Colin M Shapiro

Medical causes of insomnia—pain

Headaches
- Migraine
- Cluster headaches (stress)
- Headache of sleep apnoea
- Hypertensive, or aneurysmal
- Neck pain or injury
- Head injury

Ear, nose, and throat conditions
- Sinus infections
- Throat infections
- Croup
- Otitis

Eye diseases
- Corneal abrasions
- Acute angle glaucoma
- Flash burns, keratitis

Cardiovascular
- Angina
- Myocardial infarction
- Aortic valve disease
- Pericarditis

Gastrointestinal
- Hunger
- Hiatus hernia and hyperacidity
- Duodenal ulcer
- Gall stones and cholecystitis
- Appendicitis
- Intestinal obstruction
- Tumours

Genitourinary
- Urinary tract infections, prostatitis, and epididymitis
- Renal and ureteric stones
- Painful penile erections
- Menstrual pain

Musculoskeletal
- Mechanical neck and back strains
- Arthritis and gout
- Fibrositis/chronic fatigue
- Nocturnal leg cramps

Cancers
- Pancreas
- Bone
- Brain

Medical causes of insomnia other than pain

Nocturia
- Aging
- Infections
- Recovery from acute glomerulonephritis
- Chronic renal failure
- Tumours of the bladder and prostate

Endocrine diseases
- Diabetes with thirst, hypoglycaemia caused by insulin dose, diabetic neuropathy
- Thyroid diseases, hyperthyroidism
- Hypocalcaemia causing muscle cramps and tetany

Allergies

Asthma

Drugs

All doctors know that many medical problems present or deteriorate at night. This is not just a random event, but results from the unique physiological changes that occur during sleep. The onset of sleep can cause deterioration in illnesses that are adequately compensated for during the day, often as a result of autonomic or respiratory changes. Sleep itself may be disrupted by illness, its onset delayed and structure fragmented by problems that are bearable when the patient is awake. New techniques of measurement have led to a rapid expansion in our knowledge about the interactions between sleep and general medicine, and in this article we will focus on the most common and best understood examples.

Cardiorespiratory disorders

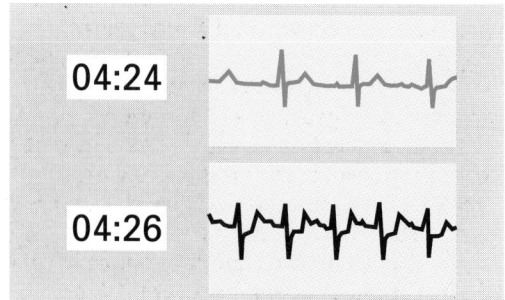

04:24

04:26

Depression of the ST segment during sleep is often asymptomatic, and does not register as arousal on the electroencephalogram.

Despite the prevalence of ischaemic heart disease nocturnal symptoms are relatively uncommon. There is a diurnal variation in the incidence of myocardial infarction that peaks between 0600 and 1200 when the patient is waking up or awake. While a patient is recovering from a myocardial infarction the quality of sleep is poor with an increased number of arousals and a reduced amount of rapid eye movement (REM) sleep. These features are common to all patients in intensive care units, and may delay recovery. There is an increased incidence of asymptomatic ST wave depression on the electrocardiogram during non-REM sleep in such patients, but the prognostic importance of these changes is not clear.

Anginal pain that is bad enough to wake the patient is more common, and can be explained by the increased myocardial consumption of oxygen as a result of increases in heart rate. When the heart rate does not change, coronary vasospasm and increased cardiac volume as a result of being supine may be responsible. Nocturnal angina is more likely to occur during non-REM sleep, and treatment is that of the underlying condition.

Medical problems during sleep

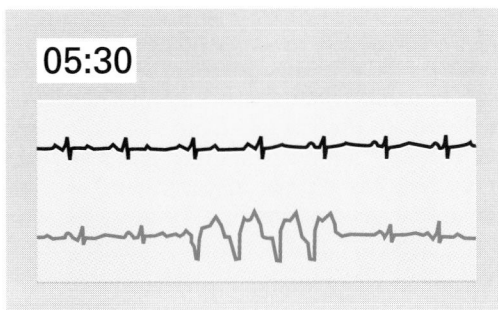

05:30

Ventricular tachycardia can occur at any time during the night in predisposed subjects.

Both heart rate and blood pressure fall during sleep, and are more variable during REM sleep probably because of the pronounced variations in parasympathetic tone that occur during REM sleep. Healthy young people can develop asymptomatic atrial and ventricular ectopic beats and even prolonged sinus arrest. Episodes of atrial fibrillation, and atrial tachycardia and flutter, occur more often during REM sleep but there is controversy about the incidence of ventricular ectopic beats and ventricular tachycardia as different groups have shown increases, reductions, or no change. Patients with coexistent lung disease have a higher incidence of arrhythmias during sleep, possibly as a result of nocturnal hypoxia and the effects of the drugs that they are taking. This group of patients commonly presents with palpitations which are worse at night (see chapter on unexpected presentations of sleep apnoea).

Breathlessness at night

- Nocturnal pulmonary oedema or bronchial asthma can cause paroxysmal nocturnal dyspnoea
- Cheyne-Stokes respiration in patients with chronic cardiac failure results in daytime lethargy and exhaustion
- Patients with severe obstructive airways disease (FEV_1 less than 1 litre) have severely disturbed sleep. Domiciliary oxygen at night is successful

Paroxysmal nocturnal dyspnoea is a classic symptom. Nocturnal pulmonary oedema or bronchial asthma can cause this, although pink, frothy sputum is seen only in patients with severe cardiac disease. Lesser degrees of pulmonary oedema are important causes of disturbed sleep, and loss of sympathetic tone during the day and absorption of oedema fluid when supine contribute to this. Subjective improvement in the quality of sleep is a good guide to the success of medical treatment.

Cheyne-Stokes respiration in patients with chronic cardiac failure is a grave prognostic sign. It is a form of central apnoea that is common during sleep among this group of patients and the resulting disruption of sleep leads to lethargy and exhaustion during the day. Recent evidence has suggested that in selected patients this can be reversed by continuous positive airway pressure ventilation (CPAP), and this also improves cardiac function during the day. Whether this has more general application we do not know.

Patients with severe chronic obstructive airways disease whose forced expiratory volume in one second (FEV_1) is less than 1 litre have severely disturbed sleep. The "pink puffers" fare worse than the "blue bloaters." In patients in the latter group the daytime hypoxia worsens during REM sleep and exacerbates their pulmonary hypertension. Domiciliary oxygen given at night abolishes this effect, improves the quality of their sleep, and may explain the improved survival among those so treated.

Gastrointestinal disorders

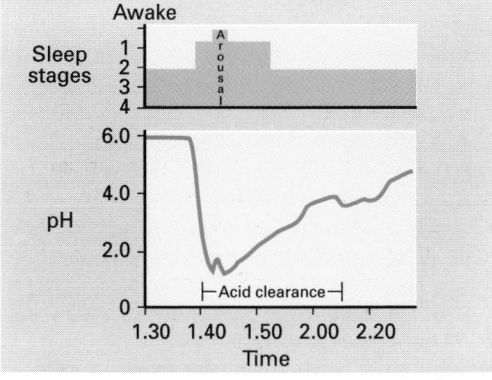

Nocturnal monitoring of oesophageal pH showing episodes of acid reflux that registered as arousals on the electroencephalogram. Unexplained nocturnal coughing is often associated with a low pH and can be treated effectively with H_2 antagonists.

Diarrhoea during the day can be incapacitating, but it seldom disrupts sleep unless there is laxative abuse or a neuropathic problem. In contrast, the upper gastrointestinal tract is particularly vulnerable to changes in parasympathetic activity during sleep. Acid secretion has a pronounced diurnal variation and waking during the night with epigastric pain is a prominent feature of untreated peptic ulceration and used to be a signal that an operation was required. Suppression of nocturnal acid secretion promotes more rapid and complete healing of ulcers. Continuous monitoring of oesophageal pH has suggested that there are two forms of oesophageal reflux; by day when the patient is erect reflux is mainly postprandial and clearance from the lower oesophagus is rapid, whereas at night, when the patient is supine, reflux clears much more slowly. Postprandial pH, and the frequency of swallowing and the volume of saliva (both of which are reduced during sleep), all affect the severity of the symptoms.

The association between nocturnal episodes of reflux and attacks of asthma remains controversial, but some patients who present with coughing at night respond to antireflux treatment.

Medical problems during sleep
Other symptoms that disrupt sleep

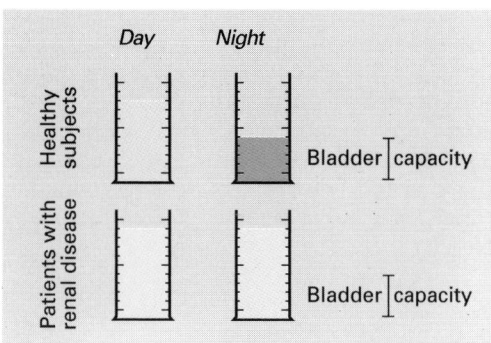

Urinary concentrating mechanisms are impaired early in some renal diseases, and cause nocturia.

Nocturia is common. The normal diurnal renal concentrating mechanism ensures reduced production of urine during the night, but this is the first function of the kidney to be affected by chronic glomerular and medullary disease. Osmotic (as a result of a high blood sugar concentration) or pharmacological (with a loop diuretic such as frusemide) diuresis has a similar effect. Factors that restrict bladder capacity range from irritable bladder caused by lower urinary tract infection to chronic distension with prostatic outflow obstruction, and can also cause nocturia. Diagnostic dip stick testing is both inexpensive and useful.

Chronic pain, be it arthritic, neoplastic, or postoperative, can affect the quality of sleep by delaying its onset, reducing the quantity of restorative slow wave sleep, and fragmenting sleep architecture. The resulting poor sleep increases the impact of the pain the next day. Disturbed sleep is an important feature of fibromyositis, and may be one of the non-specific symptoms of "myalgic encephalomyelitis" in which pain is not a feature.

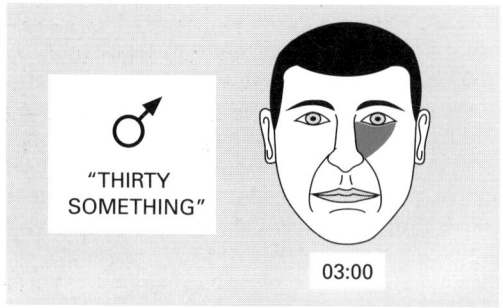

Cluster headaches occur mainly in men and in the early hours of the morning, and will wake the patient from sleep. The aetiology is thought to resemble that of migraine, but the variations in presentation are unexplained.

"Cluster" headaches are an exception to the rule that most headaches are relieved by sleep and do not disturb its quality. A typical cluster headache affects the area over one eye and wakes the patient in the early hours of the morning. It is associated with a blocked nose, running eyes, and periorbital swelling. The aetiology is unknown but attacks are commoner in men, and the clusters last from three to six weeks with freedom from symptoms in between. Prophylaxis with ergotamine or pizotifen is helpful.

Epilepsy at night is a serious problem, and may be the only time that some patients have attacks.

Other medical problems that occur at night

> These examples emphasise the importance of understanding the unique features of sleep in the practice of general medicine and confirm the need to inquire about sleep related symptoms and the quality of sleep in the routine assessment of illness. In many cases there is a close interaction between the quality of sleep and the process of the disease.

Serious medical problems can occur during sleep without the patient developing any symptoms. There is considerable controversy about the importance of some forms of hypertension during sleep. Sleep apnoea is associated with mild to moderate systemic hypertension, and people who snore are more likely to be hypertensive than those who do not. Recent studies, however, show that hypertension is not usually caused by breathing difficulties at night.

In contrast, pulmonary hypertension resulting from chronic obstructive airways disease does worsen during REM sleep, and kyphoscoliosis predisposes to nocturnal hypoventilation and hypoxia. Relief of these problems with nocturnal positive pressure ventilation can produce considerable improvements in the daytime exercise tolerance and wellbeing of patients with kyphoscoliosis.

Central sleep apnoea during REM sleep may be an independent marker of deterioration in patients with neuromuscular diseases such as Duchenne muscular dystrophy.

NOCTURNAL ASTHMA

J R Catterall, Colin M Shapiro

> I have omitted to mention this, that my fits never feize me but in the Night, and then awake me with a heavinefs, and fo grow worfe and worfe immediately.
>
> (Written by Dr (later Sir) John Floyer, himself asthmatic, in *A Treatise of the Asthma*, 1698)

Attacks of bronchial asthma are common during the night. In a recent survey in general practice of over 7000 asthmatic patients, 48% woke every night with asthma and 73% woke at least once a week, despite treatment. Coughing is common, and may be the only symptom.

Nocturnal asthma is potentially dangerous. There is an excess of deaths due to asthma during the night, and those patients most at risk are those whose peak flow rates fall furthest at night.

Pathogenesis

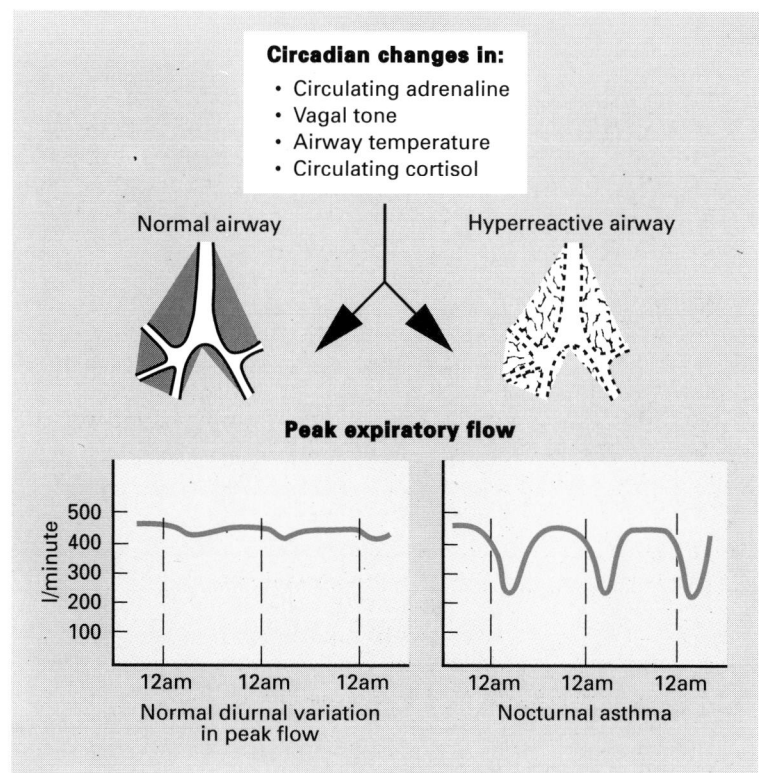

Circadian changes in:
- Circulating adrenaline
- Vagal tone
- Airway temperature
- Circulating cortisol

Normal airway — Hyperreactive airway

Peak expiratory flow

l/minute: 500 400 300 200 100

12am 12am 12am
Normal diurnal variation in peak flow

12am 12am 12am
Nocturnal asthma

The pathogenesis of nocturnal asthma.

Nocturnal asthma is a manifestation of bronchial hyper-reactivity. It is normal for the airways to narrow slightly at night, but whereas normal people have an average overnight fall in peak expiratory flow of 8% asthmatic patients have much greater falls, often in the region of 50%. The physiological changes that in normal people cause the airways to narrow at night have a greater effect on asthmatic patients because their airways are more sensitive to bronchoconstricting stimuli.

The causes of nocturnal bronchoconstriction are incompletely understood, but several factors probably coexist, including the early morning fall in circulating adrenaline, overnight changes in vagal tone and airway temperature, and circadian changes in plasma cortisol concentration. Sleep also plays a part by synchronising these circadian rhythms and REM sleep may be a trigger for bronchoconstriction (see chapter on dreams and medical illness).

Nocturnal asthma
Diagnosis

- All patients suspected of having asthma should be asked about nocturnal symptoms
- Nocturnal cough is the only symptom in some patients
- Nocturnal bronchoconstriction should be quantified by peak flow measurements at home, especially in those patients without daytime symptoms
- Nocturnal asthma is often the first indication of an exacerbation of asthma

Many asthmatic patients become so used to waking up at night that they fail to report it to the doctor. All patients who are suspected of having asthma should be asked specifically about symptoms during the night and in the early morning. Disruption of sleep has important effects on daytime performance, and children commonly complain of nightmares at times of exacerbation of asthma, as well as being irritable and having difficulties in adapting.

Whenever possible nocturnal bronchoconstriction should be confirmed and quantified by measurement of the peak flow rate at home. Reported symptoms may correlate poorly with severity and should not be relied on exclusively. There is increasing evidence that perception of bronchoconstriction varies significantly among patients.

Exacerbations of asthma

Nocturnal asthma is often the first indication of an exacerbation. Diurnal swings in the peak flow rate become less severe as the exacerbation resolves.

Absence of signs and symptoms during the day

A patient with serious symptoms during the night and early hours of the morning may have no signs or symptoms, and a normal peak flow rate, when examined at 0900. Monitoring of the peak flow rate at home is particularly useful in these patients.

Nocturnal cough

Nocturnal cough is the only symptom in some patients, particularly children. The diagnosis is not always easy to confirm by monitoring the peak flow rate, but most patients respond to a therapeutic trial of inhaled or oral corticosteroids. Any patient who has a nocturnal cough that persists for four weeks should have a chest radiograph.

"Cardiac" asthma

Paroxysmal nocturnal dyspnoea in a young person is more likely to be caused by asthma than by left ventricular failure. It is, however, common for asthma to present late in life, often with nocturnal wheeze.

Children

Recurrent nocturnal wheeze, cough, or dyspnoea in a child is caused by asthma unless proved otherwise. Isolated attacks, however, may have many causes, including infection or an inhaled foreign body.

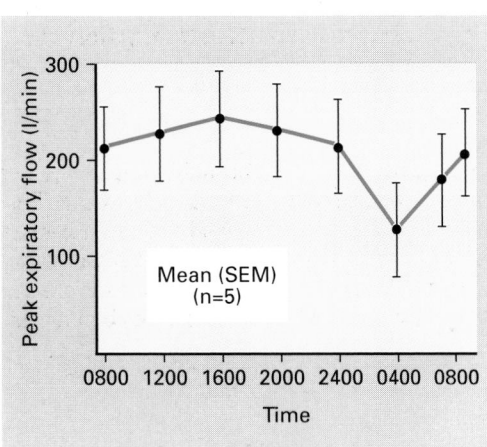

Peak flow measurements can be used to confirm the diagnosis of nocturnal asthma, to assess response to treatment, and to guide changes in treatment. An overnight fall of 15% or more from the baseline measurement is usually abnormal.

Underlying cause

Nocturnal bronchoconstriction will occur whenever there is bronchial hyper-reactivity, irrespective of the underlying cause. In occupational asthma, for example, nocturnal bronchoconstriction may be more severe than bronchoconstriction at work, and it may persist for several nights after removal of the cause. Unless a careful history is taken the nocturnal symptoms may obscure the association with work. Similarly, nocturnal symptoms that develop after a viral upper respiratory tract infection probably indicate a temporary post-infective episode of bronchial hyper-reactivity and do not necessarily mean that the patient will develop lifelong asthma.

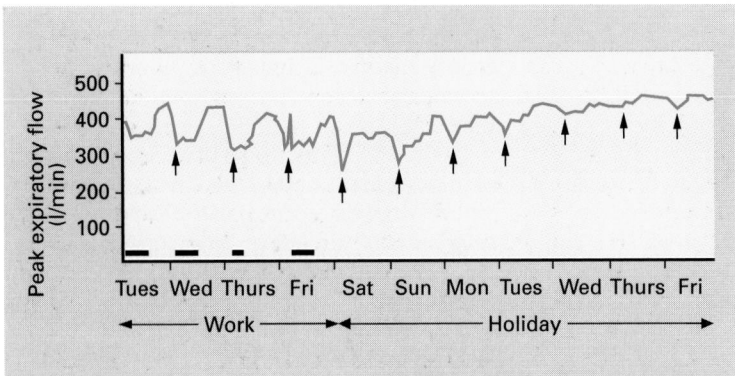

Peak expiratory flow measurements in a 39 year old man with asthma induced by exposure to isocyanate. The arrows indicate the peak flow rates on waking and the bars the period of exposure to isocyanate. The nocturnal falls in peak flow took several days to resolve after exposure to isocyanate ceased and initially obscured the association with work.

Treatment

> In general good control of asthma during the day will mean good control of asthma at night

Occasionally (in occupational asthma, or when a single removable allergen is the cause) the trigger of the bronchial hyper-reactivity can be identified and removed, but most people require drugs.

Inhaled anti-inflammatory drugs

Corticosteroids inhaled regularly are the mainstay of treatment. They reduce bronchial hyper-reactivity by suppressing inflammation of the airways. Response to treatment should be assessed by measuring the peak flow rate on waking every morning and the dose should be increased every two to three weeks until nocturnal symptoms resolve and the morning peak flow rate is within the reference range. Large doses should be delivered through a large volume spacer or a breath-actuated device for delivering dry powder. This will increase delivery to the lungs and reduce local side effects.

Other prophylactic drugs are less effective in nocturnal asthma. Sodium cromoglycate and nedocromil sodium may, however, be helpful in patients with mild symptoms and in patients who cannot tolerate large doses of inhaled corticosteroids.

Inhaled bronchodilators

The recent introduction of long acting inhaled bronchodilators has been an important development in the management of nocturnal asthma. These bronchodilators have the advantage over conventional inhaled β agonists and anticholinergic drugs that they are active throughout the night while retaining a lower risk of systemic effects than oral drugs. They should be used in addition to inhaled corticosteroids when corticosteroids alone are insufficient.

Long acting oral bronchodilators

In general inhaled bronchodilators are preferable to oral ones as the same bronchodilator effect can be achieved with smaller doses. However, oral treatment is indicated: (a) in patients whose nocturnal asthma remains uncontrolled despite high doses of inhaled steroids and inhaled bronchodilators, and (b) in young children and in others incapable of using any inhaler device—for example, because of arthritis, involuntary movements, or mental disability.

In patients whose asthma remains uncontrolled despite maximal inhaled treatment, oral theophylline is the drug of choice since it has a different mode of action from the inhaled bronchodilators which can often give additional bronchodilatation. The dose should be adjusted according to plasma or saliva concentrations. In patients who are unable to use inhalers oral β agonists are usually the first choice as they have a safer therapeutic index than theophylline and disturb sleep less.

Children

Aged 5 years or more—Children who are old enough to use an inhaler should be treated in the same way as adults. Inhaled corticosteroids are more effective than sodium cromoglycate for nocturnal asthma.

Aged 18 months-5 years—Children who are unable to use an inhaler can take inhaled drugs through a mask attached to a large volume spacer or through the bottom of a plastic cup, but these methods demand cooperation and the efficacy varies from child to child. Nebulised bronchodilators taken before bed are helpful, but their action will not last all night. Controlled release β agonists and theophylline are available in paediatric formulations, but many children prefer syrups, which, like inhaled drugs, last only a short time.

Aged less than 18 months—Nocturnal asthma is difficult to treat in this age group. Children with mild symptoms require no treatment and the parents should be reassured. For those with more troublesome symptoms a β agonist or theophylline syrup should be tried followed if necessary by a trial of a nebulised β agonist with or without ipratropium. A distressed child who fails to respond should be admitted to hospital.

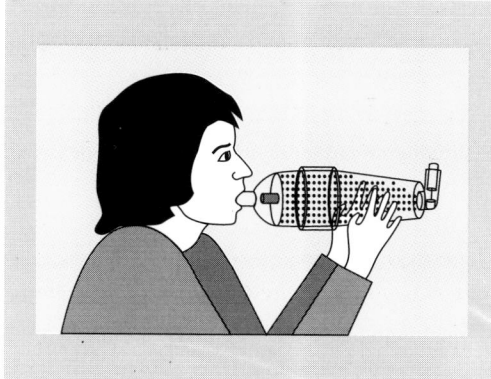

Inhaled corticosteroids are the treatment of choice for nocturnal asthma, and should be taken either from a pressurised aerosol or a dry powder inhaler. Inhaled corticosteroids from a pressurised aerosol are more effective and less likely to cause local side effects when they are taken through a large volume spacer.

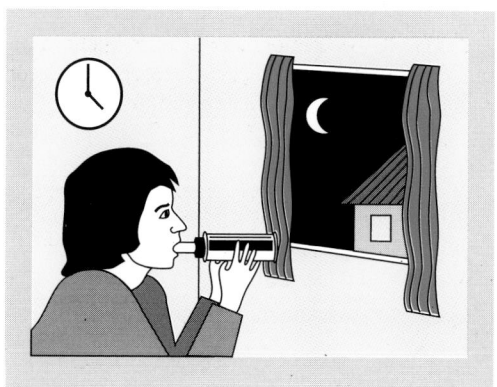

Patients should measure their peak flow whatever time they wake with asthma.

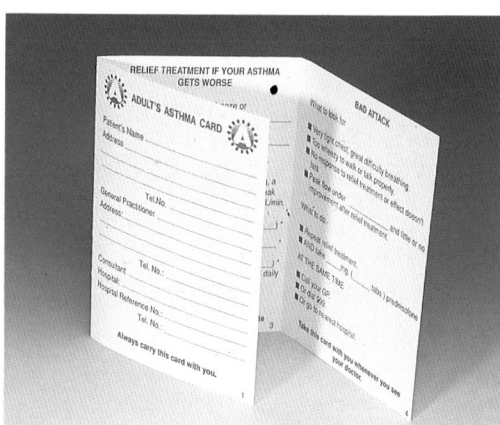

Individual self management plans constructed with a doctor or experienced nurse can improve control of asthma, including nocturnal asthma. Cards are available from the National Asthma Campaign.

Nocturnal asthma

Peak flow rate	Action
>70% of target	Continue maintenance treatment
50-70% of target	Double dose of inhaled corticosteroids
<50% of target	Start course of oral prednisolone
<150-200 l/minute	Seek medical help urgently

Self management of asthma based on morning peak expiratory flow measurements made on waking. The target peak expiratory flow is either the predicted value or the maximum consistent value achieved by the patient when well, whichever is the more appropriate.

Emergency treatment

Severe nocturnal asthma should be treated with nebulised bronchodilators and oral corticosteroids. As in any acute attack of asthma admission to hospital may be necessary, particularly if the patient responds poorly to treatment or if the peak flow rate is much less than usual (150 l/min in a normally relatively fit adult with asthma). Patients recovering from severe exacerbations of asthma should not usually be discharged from hospital until their morning peak flow rate is 70% of their value when well.

Self management

Control of asthma, including nocturnal asthma, can be improved greatly by giving patients firm guidelines about changes of treatment based on their symptoms or peak flow measurement, or both. A simple, convenient, and effective approach (which will control daytime as well as nocturnal asthma) is to base treatment on the morning peak flow reading.

Conclusion

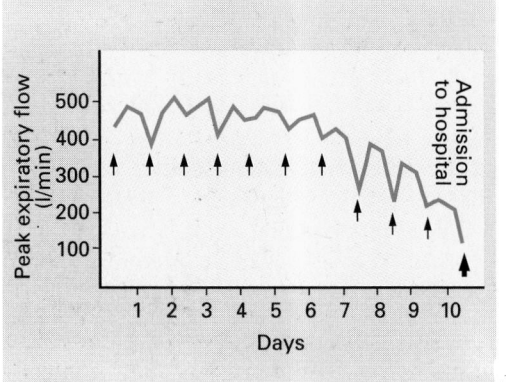

Peak expiratory flow measurements in a 27 year old man at the beginning of an acute exacerbation of asthma. The arrows indicate peak flow rates on waking. The earliest features of the exacerbation were nocturnal symptoms and a fall in the peak flow rate in the morning.

Nocturnal asthma is common and underdiagnosed, and is a sign of inadequate control of asthma. Patients who have, or are suspected of having, asthma should always be asked specifically about symptoms during the night and in the early hours, and patients with unstable asthma should be encouraged to measure their peak flow when they wake up each morning.

The treatment of choice is inhaled corticosteroids, if necessary in high doses, supplemented by inhaled bronchodilators. The development of nocturnal asthma in a patient who has not previously had nocturnal symptoms, or the worsening of pre-existing nocturnal bronchoconstriction, should be regarded as serious and indicates that the treatment should be changed.

The figure of self management of asthma is modified from Beasley R, *et al. Thorax* 1989;44:220-4, and is reproduced with permission.

SLEEP, THE IMMUNE SYSTEM, AND INFECTIOUS DISEASE

James M Krueger, Linda Toth, Colin M Shapiro

"Tir'd Nature's sweet restorer, balmy sleep!"
The complaint: night thoughts, 1742-5,
by Edward Young

There is much evidence to support the theory that sleep is a period of growth and anabolic activity, but little about the role of sleep in recovery from illness. Excessive sleep, sleepiness, fatigue, and fever are symptoms of nearly all infectious diseases and chronic inflammatory disorders. Fever probably protects during illness, but the effects of sleep are more difficult to measure. A temporal association has recently been reported in humans between the onset of sleep and the secretion of interleukin 1 and interleukin 2, which indicates that the growth and restoration that occur during sleep are part of the immune response. A study of 11 healthy men who took repeated naps during the day showed that during stage 4 sleep they had high plasma concentrations of interleukin 1 compared with when they were awake.

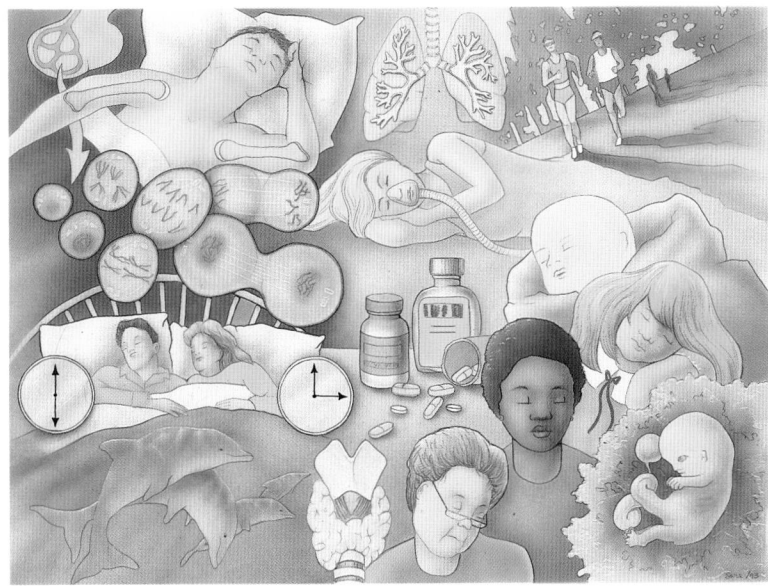

Links between anabolic activity and sleep. (By Sari O'Sullivan.)

Importance of sleep

- There is increased sleep at time of increased growth (for example, during childhood and adolescence)
- Anabolic hormones, particularly growth hormone are released during sleep
- Mytotic rates of cells increase during sleep in both nocturnal and diurnal animals
- Oxygen consumption is lower during sleep, facilitating an anabolic process
- Physiological activities (for example, exercise) and pathological disorders (for example, hyperthyroidism) which lead to increased catabolism are associated with increased slow wave sleep
- Reduced activity and metabolic turnover (for example, paraplegia and hypothyroidism) are associated with decreased slow wave sleep
- Hormones that inhibit anabolic processes (for example, corticosteroids, adrenaline, and noradrenaline are inhibited during sleep

The importance of sleep for health and recovery from disease has been recognised intuitively if not scientifically; nearly all doctors recommend that their patients should get plenty of rest and their advice is followed because that is just what the patients want to do. Whether such sleep does have any adaptive value is, however, unknown. Many disorders are associated with abnormal patterns of sleep, and the link between sleep and illness was indirectly supported by the results of a survey of over 9000 people in the United Kingdom, which showed that days of illness were positively related to deviation from the normal duration of sleep.

Many processes could contribute to the link between the immune response and sleep. For example, the circadian release of melatonin during the night is thought to counteract the immunosuppression association with glucocorticoids. Melatonin is known to regulate both the release of cytokines and cell mediated immunity.

Almost everybody is aware of the feelings of sleepiness that are associated with the onset of infectious diseases, which raises several questions:

- Does the function of sleep change after an infectious challenge?
- Does activation of the immune system affect sleep?
- Does loss of sleep affect immune functions?
- Do measures of the immune system change with sleep?
- Do sleep and the immune system share biochemical modulators?
- Does sleep in itself aid the recuperative process?

The evidence that is emerging suggests that sleep, like fever, may be a basic host defence mechanism.

Sleep, the immune system, and infectious disease
Sleep during infections

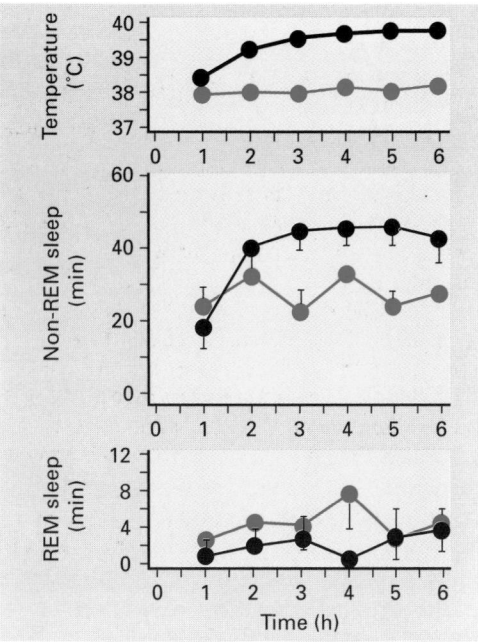

Staphylococcus aureus was fed to primary cultures of murine microglia, which digested them and released muramyl peptides (the building blocks of bacterial cell walls) into the incubation media. Fractions of the media were injected into rabbits to test the sleep promoting ability of these peptides.
Dark circles=after injection of extracts.
Light circles=control data from the same rabbits.

Although there have been no systematic studies in humans after an infective challenge, we know from recent animal studies that infections are associated with complex changes in sleep. The first studies were carried out in rabbits that were challenged with *Staphylococcus aureus* given intravenously; they showed biphasic sleep responses. Non-rapid eye movement (non-REM) sleep was greatly enhanced for about a day, and this was followed by a reduction in non-REM sleep for a further day. In most of the rabbits, particularly those with a good prognosis, there was a net gain in the amount of non-REM sleep; the increase in the amount of sleep on the first day was greater than the amount lost on the second day. In contrast, REM sleep (which occupies a much smaller amount of time in rabbits than humans), was greatly inhibited by infection with *S aureus*. In addition, electroencephalographic slow wave amplitudes increase in time with the changes in non-REM sleep. Electroencephalographic δ wave amplitudes indicate the intensity (quality) of non-REM sleep, and the changes suggest that the animals first went through a stage of very deep sleep followed by lighter sleep on the second day. The timing of the sleep responses seemed to be unrelated to the course of the fever, which started about the same time as the increase in non-REM sleep on the first day but which persisted for the second day of the experiment. The increase in neutrophils and reduction in lymphocytes also persisted, indicating that the animals remained ill throughout.

Other infective agents including Gram negative bacteria, fungi, viruses, and protozoa have also been used to challenge rabbits. The general picture of an initial increase in the amount of non-REM sleep followed by a reduction in the amount of REM sleep was usually seen, but the timing of the responses depended on the infective agent used. The route by which the rabbits were infected also influenced the timing of the effects on sleep.

Sleep loss and sleep deprivation

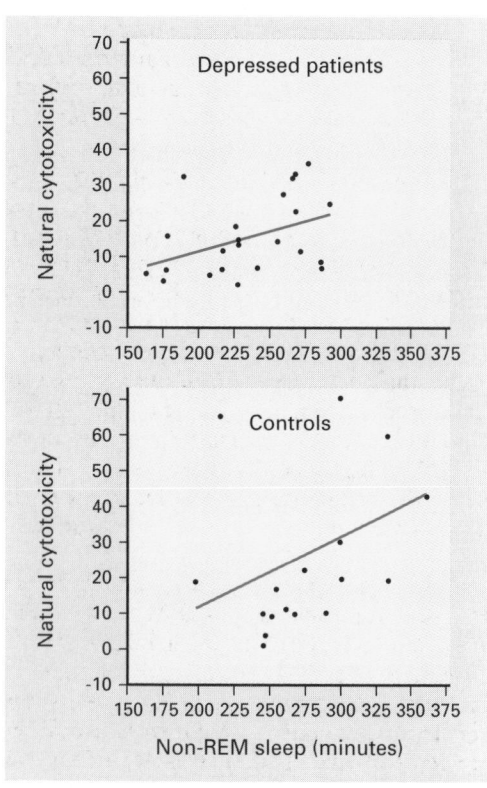

Correlations between cytotoxicity of natural killer cells and non-REM sleep in depressed patients (n=23) and control subjects (n=17) (r=0·51, p<0·01).

Research workers in Chicago deprived rats of sleep for long periods; eventually the rats died. It has recently been shown that rats that are deprived of sleep (but not matched controls) develop septicaemia, which seems to be the probable cause of death, so loss of sleep does in some way adversely affect an animal's ability to defend itself against microbial invasion.

There are few studies of the interaction between sleep deprivation and immunity in humans. In one, 20 young adults (21-30 years old) were deprived of sleep for 64 hours, and they all showed increases in monocytes, granulocytes, and natural killer (NK) cells, and in the activity of NK cells.

Another study in which nine healthy women (mean age 36 years) were allowed to sleep between 0300 and 0700, or between 2100 and 0100, showed that they had a 25%-30% reduction in the activity of NK cells. The authors concluded that even a moderate disturbance of sleep imposed by a night of partial sleep deprivation seemed to produce a reduction in NK activity. A night of recovery sleep restored levels of NK activity to baseline values.

A reduction in cellular immunity in humans was shown in two other reports: in the first patients showed reduced proliferation of lymphocytes in response to stimulation with phytohaemagglutinin, and in the other the activity of NK cells was reduced after 40 hours awake. Limited sleep loss (insomnia) has also been associated with a reduction in activity of NK cells. In a study of 23 depressed patients and 17 control subjects total time asleep, duration of non-REM sleep, and sleep efficiency all correlated with the activity of NK cells. The large number of publications that comment on the suppression of immune reactivity in depressed patients may be referring to the disruption of sleep that occurs during periods of depression.

If we tentatively accept the conclusion that loss of sleep adversely affects host defences and may even lead to disease, then it seems reasonable to propose that under normal conditions at least some aspects of host defence are linked to sleep states. These results all seem to support the idea that rest helps our defences against infection.

Mechanisms of interaction between sleep and immunity

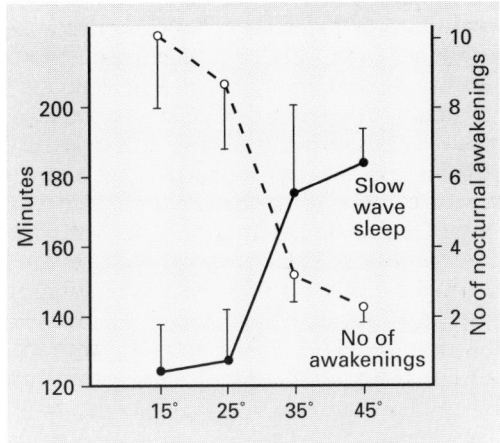

Mean total slow wave sleep (min) and total number of awakenings in 11 subjects on each night after exposure to four different temperatures for four hours ending 1·5 hours before the onset of sleep.

Some evidence for the role of interleukin 1 in the physiological regulation of sleep

- Interleukin 1β enhances sleep in rats, rabbits, and cats
- Anti-interleukin 1β antibodies inhibit non-REM sleep in rabbits
- Substances that induce interleukin 1 production—for example, muramyl peptides—enhance sleep
- Substances that inhibit interleukin 1 production inhibit sleep (for example, prostaglandin E$_2$)
- Patients receiving treatment with interferon report excessive sleepiness
- Interleukin 1 mRNA is in normal brain and other physiological tissues such as cerebrospinal fluid, milk, and plasma
- There are neurons with interleukin 1-like immunoactivity in human and rat anterior hypothalamus
- Plasma concentrations of interleukin 1 peak in humans at the onset of non-REM sleep
- Interleukin 1 concentrations in cerebrospinal fluid vary in phase with sleep/wake cycles
- Interleukin 1 interacts with the β aminobutyric acid (GABA$_A$) receptor; the GABA$_A$ receptor is involved in diazepam altered sleep

Thermoregulation

We are beginning to understand the interaction of sleep and thermoregulation, and the humoral regulation of both the immune response and sleep. Exposure to heat before sleep increases the amount of slow wave sleep, but with extreme amounts of heat the subsequent sleep pattern is disturbed. If a heat stress is applied to a normal sleeping subject, the total amount of slow wave sleep is reduced. Some studies have shown that there is a progressive fall in temperature during each episode of slow wave sleep, which is particularly pronounced during the first two sleep cycles, but it is not clear whether the temperature rhythms are causing the changes in slow wave sleep, or whether the slow wave sleep is facilitating the drop in temperature which starts before the onset of sleep. The relationship is further complicated by the fact that responses to fever induced by bacteria can be blocked without affecting sleep responses, and some pyrogenic peptides inhibit sleep while others promote it. The interaction between control of temperature, sleep, and immune responses requires further elucidation, but interestingly it is at the extremes of life when circadian sleep rhythms and temperature rhythms are less clear that there is greater vulnerability to infection.

Role of biological molecules

Several molecules play a part in the regulation of sleep and immune processes. Muramyl peptides that are produced by macrophages from phagocytosed bacterial cell walls activate macrophages to produce modifiers of the immune response. Other products of bacterial cell walls (for example, endotoxin) and certain viral products (for example, viral double-standard RNA) also increase the length of sleep and the production of modifiers of the immune response, one class of which are called cytokines. Cytokines are concerned with the amplification, coordination, and regulation of the immune response; some are also produced in the brain and respond to infection or injury of the central nervous system. They probably also play a part in sleep responses to systemic infection—for example, intravenous injection of cytokines will induce many central responses including increased sleep. Specific cytokines known to affect sleep include interleukin 1$_\alpha$, interleukin 1$_\beta$, tumour necrosis factor α, and interferon alfa.

The hypothesis that cytokines have a role in physiological processes is controversial. The hypothesis is that, under normal conditions, low basal production of cytokines and their effects vary in subtle ways with one or more physiological processes. The specificity of the response for any one physiological function—for example, sleep—would arise from a network of several cytokines and hormones with interacting multiple neuronal sets, each having a different array of sensitivities to different cytokines and hormones. After pathological disturbances the production of one or more cytokines would be greatly increased through microbial (or other) stimuli in a site-specific way. This would then induce disease in a way similar to those produced by excessive production of hormones. Interleukin 1$_\beta$ is the only cytokine that has been studied extensively as regards its effects on sleep, and there is a lot of evidence that strongly implicates it in the physiological regulation of sleep.

Other cytokines also have a role in the regulation of sleep and its response to infection. Tumour necrosis factor α promotes non-REM sleep in rabbits, and anti-tumour necrosis factor antibodies inhibit sleep in rats. Sleep deprivation as well as infection increase systemic production of tumour necrosis factor. Similarly, interferon alfa$_2$ promotes non-REM sleep in both rabbits and rats. Patients who are undergoing treatment with interferon complain of sleepiness. Sleep deprivation and other stressors increase the ability of immunocytes to produce interferon. Despite such promising data, however, our understanding of the regulation of cytokines in the brain concerning sleep is severely limited, though these data do emphasise the close association between sleep and immune regulation.

Sleep, the immune system, and infectious disease
Sleep and AIDS

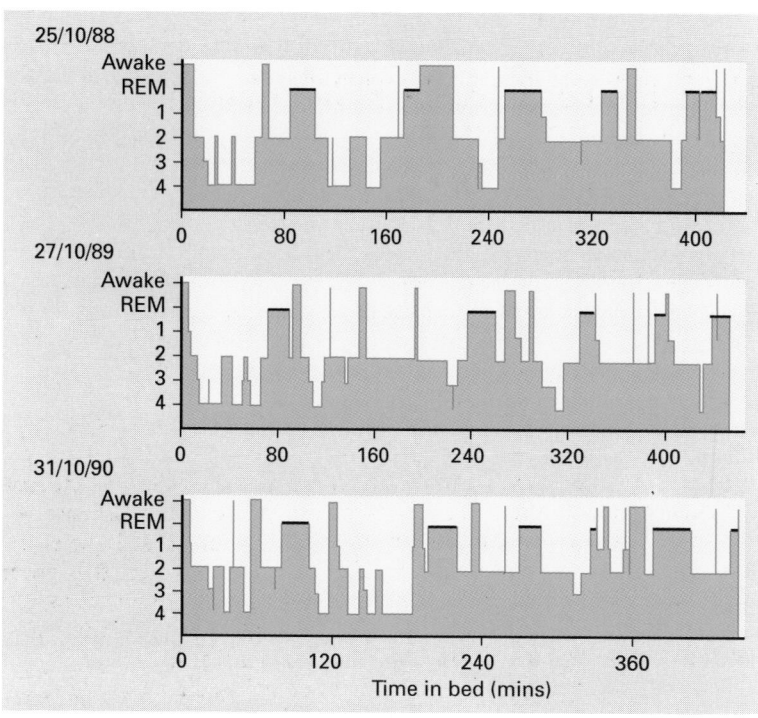

Changes in sleep pattern as AIDS progresses.

The link between immune dysfunction and sleep is emphasised by the changes in sleep that follow infection with HIV. A prospective study of 112 homosexual men, 62 of whom were HIV positive, showed that the ones who were seropositive slept more, napped more, and had reduced alertness in the morning. A study of 14 patients infected with HIV and 10 age matched control subjects who were not infected showed that after infection there is a loss of normal sleep architecture, and more slow wave sleep occurs late in the night with more REM sleep occuring early in the night.

In a study of 15 patients with AIDS and 15 age matched control subjects, all night sleep recordings showed with a spectral analysis technique that there was less consistency between the two hemispheres in the patients with AIDS. The same authors showed that the severity of illness correlated with the flattening of the distribution of REM sleep throughout the night. In a third study of men infected with HIV, the authors concluded that "sleep disturbances occur in the course of HIV infection and suggest that the observed alterations of sleep physiology may be a consequence of central nervous system involvement and/or immune defence mobilisation in the early phases of HIV infection."

Conclusion

> Rest is part of the host's defence against infection

One of the important questions to ask is: does sleep itself help us to recuperate from infection? Though we have no absolute answer, indirect evidence suggests that it does. After either a bacterial or a fungal challenge the specific sleep pattern that develops is related to the clinical response of the animal, and the more favourable the prognosis the more prolonged and intense is the non-REM sleep after the challenge. Increased sleep, like temperature, may be beneficial during infection.

The data that we have reinforce our intuitive belief that sleep is altered by infection and has some sort of non-specific beneficial role in recovery of the host. Little attention has been paid to these issues until recently, and whether any useful treatment will result from this attention is not yet clear. What is important is that these studies are leading to a new understanding of how sleep is regulated and to what its function is.

The illustration by Sari O'Sullivan is reproduced with permission of the artist.

SLEEP PROBLEMS IN PATIENTS WITH MEDICAL ILLNESS

Colin M Shapiro, Gerald M Devins, M R G Hussain

Sleep complaints are ubiquitous in patients with medical illness. A recent survey of outpatients attending hospital clinics indicated that the vast majority of patients reported sleep disruption concomitant with their condition. The proportion with complaints ($>70\%$) was more than twice that among control subjects. Doctors rarely ask about sleep problems in the context of medical illness despite the fact that the patient's first complaint may be that a particular symptom caused sleep disruption.

There are specific reasons for sleep disruptions in patients with medical illness—for example, people are often deprived of sleep before an operation. Polysomnography has shown that there is a preoperative reduction in slow wave sleep and that this is related to the anticipated importance of surgery. The increase in deep sleep that occurs after an operation is thought to facilitate the healing process.

A variety of sleep variables may be influenced by specific disorders and particular treatments and each of these effects is likely to differ. A decrease in deep (slow wave) sleep, for example, may lead to a sensation of having low energy, whereas repeated interruption of sleep may lead to daytime sleepiness.

Drugs may also disrupt sleep architecture by suppressing rapid eye movement (REM) sleep or by causing a withdrawal effect during the night. In both cases the drug clearly alters sleep, but the impact on health and recovery may differ.

Fatigue is common in several medical conditions. Clinicians, researchers, and patients themselves claim that the fatigue experienced in certain medical conditions differs qualitatively from the experience of tiredness or sleepiness. However, there have been few attempts to separate these states. In this article we provide an overview of the impact of medical disorders on sleep.

Factors that may indicate a disruption of sleep architecture in medically ill patients

- Movement arousals (number)
- Frequent changes in sleep stage (per hour of sleep)
- Awakenings in first six hours of sleep (number)
- Sleep efficiency (%)
- Apnoea index
- Leg kicks (total number)
- Abnormal REM latency
- Reduced slow wave sleep corrected for age (% below normal)
- Total sleep time
- Long awakenings (10 min)
- α Pattern on electroencephalogram

Sleep problems in specific conditions

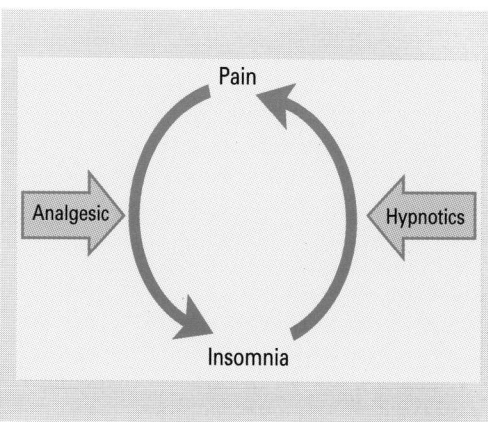

Although sleep related problems among medically ill patients have only recently begun to be investigated, there is a rapidly growing body of evidence that sleep can be profoundly affected by ill health.

End stage renal disease

Several studies have examined sleep disturbances among patients with end stage renal disease, in which sleep is significantly altered. Patients receiving renal replacement therapy by maintenance haemodialysis or peritoneal dialysis have considerably more severe sleep disorders compared with healthy controls. Patients receiving dialysis commonly complain of insomnia and daytime fatigue. However, the factors responsible for these problems remain to be elucidated. We could speculate that night time sleep problems might be attributable to the immobilisation imposed by maintenance haemodialysis and the propensity of patients to nap during treatment as a result, but no differences have been observed between the night time sleep characteristics of patients treated by haemodialysis as

Sleep problems in patients with medical illness

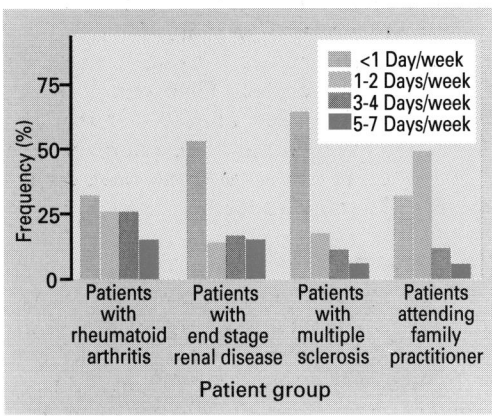

Frequency of restless sleep across four patient groups.

compared with peritoneal dialysis. In one study caffeine intake and worry were the only factors associated with reported sleep disturbance in renal disease; Kt/V values did not predict reported sleep problems.

Patients with end stage renal disease can have some of the most intractable sleep difficulties, which do not easily respond to treatment. Profound sleep disturbances are commonly the result of sleep related periodic involuntary limb movements that occur at 20-40 second intervals, leading to a disruption of the continuity of sleep. These disruptions compromise sleep quality, which is different from the sleep problems in other conditions (see below).

Psychosocial factors also seem to be related to sleep disturbances in patients with end stage renal disease. It has been shown, for example, that patients receiving dialysis who report increased tiredness and sleep disturbance also report increased negative affect. These observations must be qualified, however, by the finding that the patients who experience sleep disturbances seem to lack insight into the problem. One study concluded that use of denial as a coping defence may decrease awareness of sleep dysfunction in end stage renal disease.

Increased insomnia coupled with increased self-administration of hypnotic drugs is often the forerunner of a worsening clinical state in patients receiving maintenance dialysis. Recent research on sleep problems and myocardial infarction showed a parallel finding: an increase in insomnia predicted increased risk of myocardial infarction two weeks later.

Comparison of features in chronic fatigue syndrome and fibromyalgia

Features	Chronic fatigue syndrome	Fibromyalgia
Symptoms and signs:		
Fatigue	+++ (97%)	++ (90%)
Pain	+	++
Sleep disturbance	+	+
α Pattern on electroencephalogram	+ ve	+ ve
Decreased slow wave sleep	?	+
Depression	✓	✓
Tender points*	+	++
Other physical symptoms (such as paresthesias)	+/−	+/−
Epidemiology		
Preponderance among women	79%	87%
Age at presentation	25-40 years	30-45 years
Weather effects	?	✓
Comorbid diagnosis (for example, irritable bowel syndrome, premenstrual syndrome)	Common	Common
Evolution		
Sociocultural		
"Workaholism"	✓	✓
Masked depression	✓	✓
Western disease	✓	✓
Participation in self help groups	++	?
Relapse triggered or precipitated by stress	✓	✓
No definitive investigations	True	True
Pathology delineated	No	No
Treatment response		
Cognitive therapy	Yes	Yes
Low dose antidepressants	Improve sleep and muscular symptoms	Improve sleep and muscular symptoms
High dose antidepressants	Improve comorbid mood disturbance	Improve comorbid mood disturbance
Improved sleep (for example, with cyclopyrrolone)	Yes (anecdotal)	Yes
Exercise treatment	+/−	+/−
Light therapy	?	?

*Mean (SD) tenderpoint scores are as follows: 3·5 (2·6) in normal people; 16·9 (14·1) in those with chronic fatigue syndrome; 33·0 (11·8) in those with fibromyalgia.
+/− = May be present; ✓=Present but no degrees; ?=Uncertain.

Rheumatoid arthritis

Middle insomnia (that is, fragmented sleep) is associated with exacerbations of illness in patients with rheumatoid arthritis. Patients with fragmented sleep experienced increased fatigue and joint pain. This is consistent with findings in animals and humans that sleep deprivation reduces the pain threshold. Indeed, in one study, 70% of arthritic patients took benzodiazepines to overcome night pain. These findings suggest that it is profitable to treat pain and insomnia concurrently owing to their reciprocal effects. In another study, however, pain predicted subsequent increases in sleep problems in rheumatoid arthritis but the reverse predictive relation was not also observed, endorsing the traditional view to treat the primary cause.

Fibromyalgia and the chronic fatigue syndrome

Fibromyalgia is characterised by multiple tender points and complaints of fatigue. In a recent overview the features of fibromyalgia and the chronic fatigue syndrome were found to be very similar. There is a high incidence of sleep abnormalities (67% in a recent polysomnographic study of patients with the chronic fatigue syndrome). A commonly reported feature in the sleep of these patients is an α electroencephalographic pattern. This implies that α waves, which are usually associated with relaxed wakefulness (with eyes closed), intrude into the sleep electroencephalogram. When it is explained to patients that this is an indication of poor quality sleep they often respond that they feel as if they "just skim below the surface of sleep."

Sleep problems in patients with medical illness

These patients commonly describe feeling as if they are awake during sleep and completely misjudge the duration before sleep onset and the total duration of sleep. This qualitative change in sleep may be partly responsible for the complaints of fatigue and pain often reported by patients with fibromyalgia. This example of poor sleep quality due to α intrusion is very different from the repeated interruption of sleep due to nocturnal myoclonus in end stage renal disease, as described above.

Neuromuscular conditions

Neuromuscular conditions can affect sleep profoundly. In one study, for example, 88% of patients with Parkinson's disease reported significant sleep problems. Bradykinesia during the night is especially problematic. Patients with advanced Parkinson's disease may experience sleep/wake dysfunction due to cumulative effects of motor abnormalities, neurochemical changes, depression, drugs, and dementia. Episodic muscle contractions, irregular fragmentary twitches, and jerks of the extremities may occur during light sleep. About 33% of patients with Parkinson's disease experience periodic leg movements. Vocalisations and prolonged activation of muscle tone may occur during REM sleep and may, in some cases, evolve into REM sleep behaviour disorders. Occasionally, visual hallucinations may be described and may be the consequence of sleep deprivation.

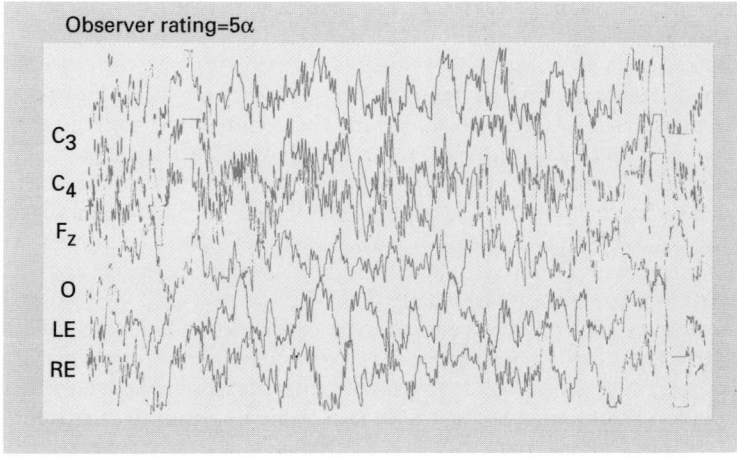

α Pattern on electroencephalogram in a patient with the chronic fatigue syndrome.

Sleep disruptions that inhibit healing

> **Aetiologic factors in the intensive care unit syndrome**
>
> - Patient's age
> - Patient's psychological history
> - Use of cardiopulmonary bypass pump
> - Metabolic and drug factors
> - Severity of illness
> - **Sleep deprivation**

> Given an adequate amount of sleep, patients in intensive care units will experience less physical and psychological stress and fewer mental status alterations and, thus, will have a more rapid and less traumatic recovery

There are many situations in which sleep may be disrupted, and this may prolong or worsen a disease process. An intensive care unit environment, with its attendant continuous lighting, noise throughout day and night, and the disruption of sleep for the purpose of investigations, is a typical example. The so called "intensive care unit syndrome" has been held responsible for inhibiting patient recovery. One associated aetiological factor is sleep deprivation. An alteration in mental state, including delusions and paranoia, has been noted with sleep deprivation, which is common in the intensive care unit setting. Recovery sleep in the experimental situation or transfer out of the intensive care unit often leads to a resolution of these symptoms.

In a German study of patients in intensive care units with neurological disorders who underwent polysomnographic monitoring, there was a pronounced reduction in REM sleep; occasionally no REM sleep was recorded. Changes in this group were related to specific neurological lesions. Patients with demyelinating diseases, such as multiple sclerosis, did not show many sleep pattern abnormalities.

In another study careful documentation of 62 subjects over their first three days in the intensive care unit showed that most (56%) were sleep deprived during the first day. This declined over time, but 20% were still judged to be sleep deprived in their third day in the unit. More severely ill patients were more sleep deprived. Patients who were sleep deprived to a comparatively greater extent were also significantly more likely to display the intensive care unit syndrome.

Several other factors which lead to a deterioration in sleep architecture in relation to the process of healing include pain, age related sleep deterioration, and the psychosocial stress associated with ill health. Drugs used in various illnesses have an impact on sleep and daytime alertness which, in some cases, may be unexpected—for example, sleep disruption attributable to hypertension may be compounded by drug effects, leading to the paradox where disruption is significantly greater in treated patients.

Sleep problems in patients with medical illness
Treating sleep problems in the context of medical illness

> **Steps in tackling fatigue in a medical condition**
>
> (1) Investigate standard medical possibilities—for example, thyroid disease—and make a diagnosis if possible. Contemplate multiple diagnoses. Query depression
>
> (2) Treat the medical illness to the extent this is possible. Give palliative treatment. Use stimulating antidepressants or electroconvulsive therapy if needed
>
> (3) Consider whether drugs contribute to the fatigue—for example, antiepileptic drugs. Can the specific drug or the dosing schedule be altered?
>
> (4) Review sleep hygiene of the patient. Even small changes in activity make a difference. Ensure that the patient does not take daytime naps or have any unnecessary nocturnal interruptions of sleep—that is, consolidate sleep and restrict bedtime to improve sleep efficiency
>
> (5) Paradoxically, a hypnotic which improves sleep may lessen daytime fatigue
>
> (6) Consider the possibility of a primary sleep disorder and investigate accordingly

There is a current trend against the use of hypnotic drugs. Particularly in the medically ill, this must be tempered insofar as improved sleep may facilitate recovery and poor sleep may lead to increasing anxiety and distress. Moreover, poor sleep may eliminate the opportunity of relief from physical symptoms.

Practical considerations must also be taken into account—for example, in chronic disabling conditions, such as Parkinson's disease, sleep disruption can be minimised by arranging for a portable commode to be placed at the bedside. Adjustments to the type, dose, or scheduling of drugs should be considered to minimise potential iatrogenic causes of insomnia. Respite admissions for the patient or advising a couple to use separate bedrooms may improve sleep quality for the spouse.

The interaction of many drugs with hypnotic drugs needs to be carefully balanced in medically ill patients.

Compliance with treatment may also be influenced by the sleep effects of non-hypnotic drugs. Impact on sleep may be the key determinant of quality of life differences across alternative treatments. In a study of patients with joint pain, for example, two treatment groups were compared in terms of quality of life. Patients treated with a combination of dextropropoxiphene and paracetamol reported a significant excess of tiredness and sleep disturbance compared with those treated with diclofenac sodium slow release but no other quality of life difference was detected.

Quality of life

> There is a reciprocal interaction between the influence of medical illnesses on sleep. Careful attention to the sleep complaints of medically ill patients will facilitate improved healing, wellbeing, and a greater ability to cope with disease. Improved compliance with treatments used in medical illnesses is promoted if sleep related issues are taken into consideration

Not surprisingly, sleep difficulties can compromise quality of life in patients with medical illness. Depression and negative affect occur, at least in part, because of the disruptions in lifestyle, activities, and interests ("illness intrusiveness") that occur as a result of illness induced reductions in energy, stamina, and cognitive arousal. Illness intrusiveness into important life domains (for example, work, family relationships, leisure, friendships) occurs with greater intensity among patients with chronic illness who experience relatively frequent episodes of restless sleep. A recent comparison of sleep problems across three chronic conditions indicated that restless sleep occurred most commonly among patients with rheumatoid arthritis, moderately commonly in those with end stage renal disease, and least commonly among people with multiple sclerosis. Moreover, the relation between restless sleep and emotional distress was mediated by illness intrusiveness—that is, restless sleep seemed to exert its impact on emotional distress through its disruption of lifestyle, activities, and interests. These relations were observed in both depressed and non-depressed patients, indicating that the phenomenon could not be attributed to a depressive response.

DREAMS AND MEDICAL ILLNESS

Mark Katz, Colin M Shapiro

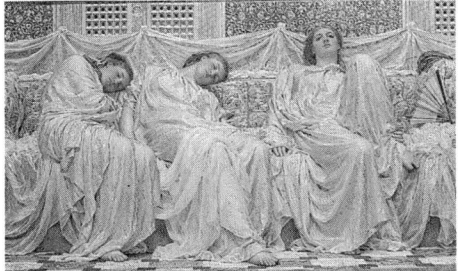

"Dreamers" by Albert Moore.

Doctors and investigators who are interested in the influence of mind over matter have long thought that dreams may reflect or influence health. The ancient Greeks, including Hippocrates and Galen, believed not only that dreams could yield both diagnostic and prognostic information, but also that they were the medium through which the gods alleviated illness. Aristotle believed that during sleep the mind received stimuli from both the external environment and from within the body, and that these served as the building blocks on which dreams were constructed. There are certain aspects of life that the mind is aware of only through the recollection and understanding of dreams.

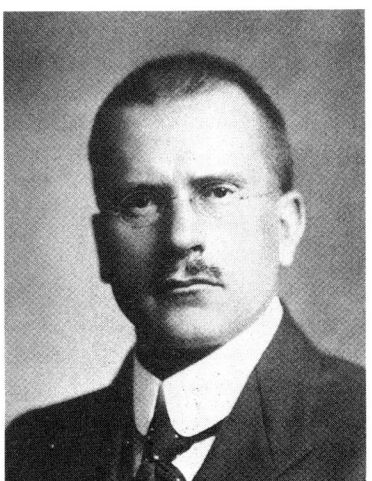

Carl Gustav Jung, 1875-1961.

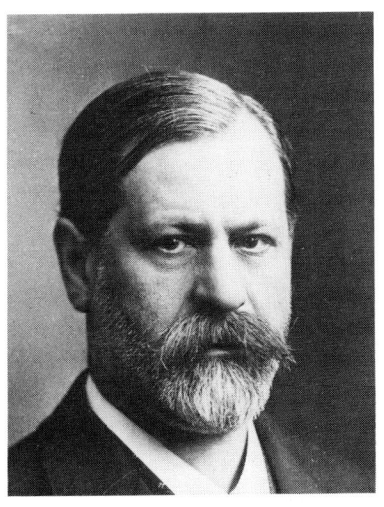

Sigmund Freud, 1856-1939.

Modern theories

Modern investigation of dreams began with Freud's classic *The Interpretation of Dreams*, which was first published in 1900. Freud believed that dreams represented unconscious wishes that were repressed because they were unacceptable. He also believed that organic states could instigate dreams—for example, patients with lung disease who dreamed of suffocation or patients with heart disease who dreamed that they died horribly.

Freud's theories were expanded by his followers. Jung believed that dreams contained unrecognised information that patients needed to understand and integrate into their consciousness, and Adler that dreams had a potential role in the solving of problems.

Link with illness

These explanations of the functions of dreams and their relation to illness were complemented by the discovery in 1953 that rapid eye movement (REM) sleep was associated with dreaming. The finding that "dream sleep" was associated with wide fluctuations in physiological measurements (including temperature, heart rate, blood pressure, gastric acid secretion, and serum catecholamine concentrations) similar to those noted during periods of stress emphasised the possibility of a link between dreaming and stress related physical illness. Until recently there have been few empirical observations and most of these have been case reports of dreams that were temporally associated with periods of illness.

Current research, however, has shown that dreams may:

* Reflect the presence of organic disease
* Cause or precipitate organic disease
* Serve as a marker for either psychological conflict or personality traits that might influence the development of organic disease (so called psychosomatic illness).

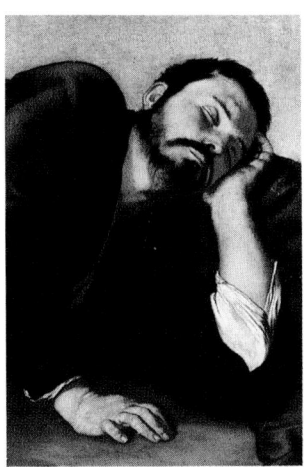

"Jacob's dream" by Jusepe de Ribera.

Dreams and medical illness
Dreams as reflectors of biological illness

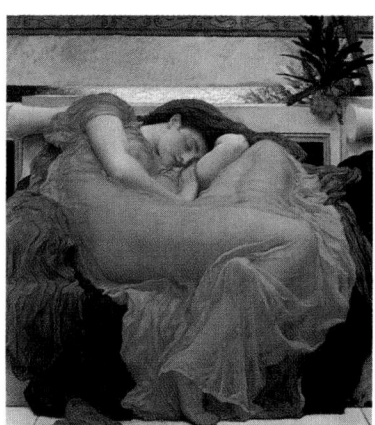

"Flaming June" by Lord Leighton.

It has long been recognised that dreams may reflect the presence of illness even if the patient is unaware of it. In particular, dreams about death and dying are prevalent among people with serious organic (especially cardiac) disease. Prospective studies have shown that among men dreams of death, and among women dreams of separation, correlate with worse clinical outcomes independent of the disease, and with the severity of cardiac dysfunction (measured by ejection fraction) in patients with cardiac disease.[1] Dreams of "lost resources" have been correlated with the finding of brain atrophy on computed tomography in elderly patients without overt signs of organic brain disease.[2] None of these findings could be related either to anticipation of a poor prognosis by the patient, or to awareness of disability.

One study reported that patients who did not dream at all had the worst prognosis (that is, the highest mortality),[3] and it has been hypothesised that dreams "warn" medically ill patients whose illness is seen as threatening to both the body and the ego[4]; when, however, the threat becomes too severe the dreams may disappear altogether.

How medical illness is reflected in dreams

Illness	Characteristic of dream
Cardiac dysfunction	Death and dying (men) Separation (women)
Brain atrophy	Lost resources
Migraine	Terror
Neurological events	Loss of recall Deficits in visual imagery Loss of narrative
Drugs (including withdrawal)	Loss of recall Vivid or bizarre
Narcolepsy	Vivid or bizarre
Severe organic disease	Ability to dream is lost

Effect of neurological damage

Changes in the amount and quality of dreaming may reflect neurological damage. Cerebrovascular events, particularly posterior parieto-occipital lesions, are associated with loss of recall and little visual content in dreams. Lesions of the right hemisphere may be associated particularly with deficits in visual imagery, whereas those in the left hemisphere may result in loss of structure and context of dream imagery.[5] Damage to the frontal lobes may result in difficulty in remembering dreams. In addition, injury to the brain, temporal lobe epilepsy, and Parkinson's disease have all been associated with disturbances in the ability to dream. Patients with narcolepsy commonly have vivid, bizarre, often frightening, dreams which are presumably related to alterations in the amount or quality of REM sleep.

Effect of drugs

Drugs may also influence the quality and extent of dreaming. Patients with Parkinson's disease who are taking levodopa may have vivid and unusual dreams. Drugs that suppress REM sleep such as antidepressants may interfere with the production of dreams, and withdrawal states that are associated with a rebound increase in the amount of REM sleep may cause disturbing dreams. These effects are seen with various substances including alcohol, benzodiazepine sedatives, and antidepressant and anxiolytic drugs.

Dreams that cause or precipitate medical illness

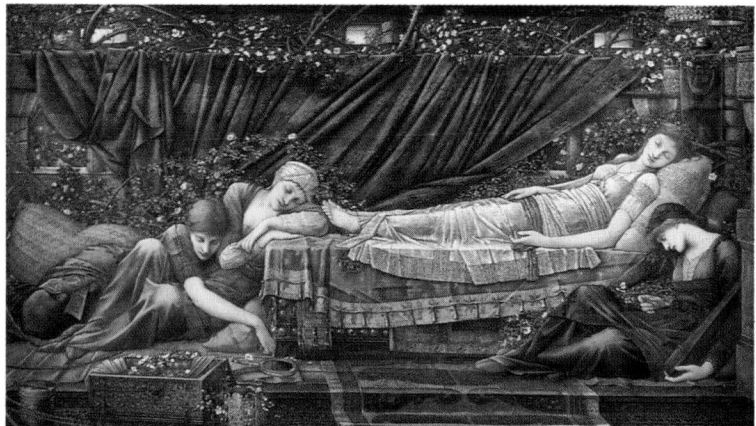

"The sleeping Beauty" by Sir Edward Burne-Jones.

Numerous physiological variables are altered during REM sleep, and there are fluctuations in the autonomic nervous and hormonal systems which have been implicated in the triggering of a number of medical events. There have been numerous case reports of cardiac disturbances (including atrial and ventricular arrhythmias, asystole, and ischaemia) after dreams, and attacks of migraine and nocturnal asthma have been associated with dreaming and REM sleep. One study, in which recall of dreams was compared after REM and non-REM sleep in asthmatic patients and age and sex matched controls, found that the differences were considerable, and more robust than the changes in respiratory function.[6] Subsequent studies indicated that the changes in breathing were related to dreams, particularly emotional ones.[7] Patients with duodenal ulcers secrete significantly more gastric acid during REM sleep than patients without, which may explain nocturnal attacks of ulcer pain.

Dreams as markers of psychosomatic illness

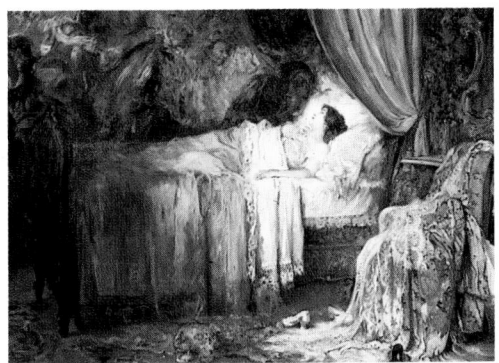

"Dreams" by Emilio Poy y Dalmau.

Dreams that indicate psychosomatic illness have been differentiated from other dreams by the presence of themes of conflict—aggression, fear, helplessness, and death. In a number of cases these dreams actually preceded the onset of a psychosomatic illness. Hypertensive patients have been differentiated from patients without hypertension by the increased amount of hostility in the dreams of hypertensive patients.

The "alexithymia construct" is a hypothesised stable personality trait that describes some people's inability to be aware of and communicate emotional states. Alexithymic people are also thought to have little or no fantasy life, impoverished dreams, and a tendency to mundane operational thinking. Their emotional states are poorly regulated and their autonomic nervous systems are persistently aroused, which predisposes them to various psychosomatic illnesses.

In patients with insomnia shorter episodes of REM sleep and increased eye movement density are related to more vivid, frightening, and disrupted dreaming.

Conclusion

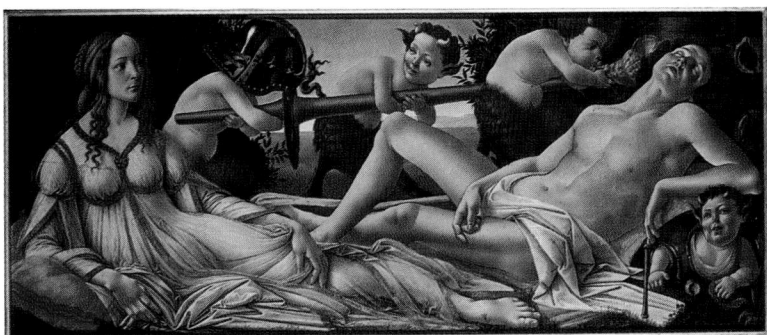

"Venus and Mars" by Botticelli.

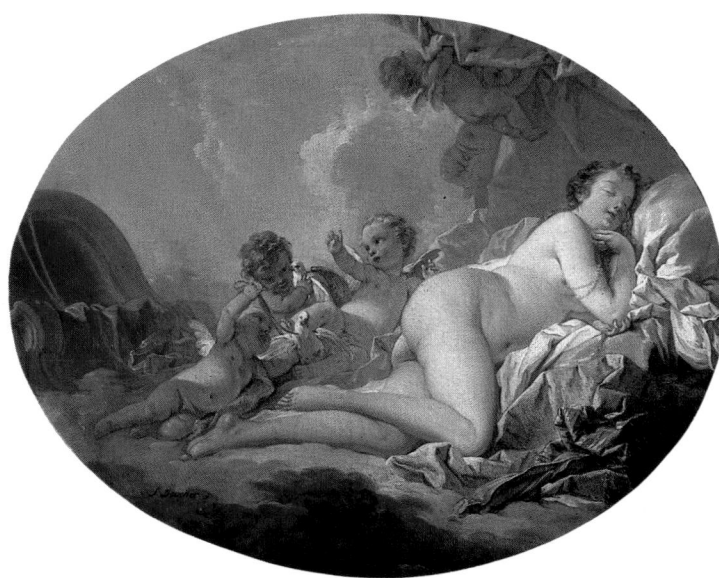

"The sleeping Venus" by Francois Boucher.

Dreams may reflect underlying organic disease, and are occasionally the first clue that the disease is present. Alterations in the function of the autonomic nervous system during REM sleep may trigger various organic illnesses. It is not certain that the emotional content of dreams is the precipitating factor, but studies of the content of dreams and bronchial function in asthmatic patients indicate that it is.

Suppression of dreams in ill people may be an adaptive defence mechanism (for example, in asthmatic patients no REM sleep=no dreams= no bronchoconstriction). Conversely, it may be a reflection of neurological disease or a sign of severe organic dysfunction.

The study of dreams detected in the laboratory by polysomnography—that is, waking subjects during REM sleep—provides opportunities to test specific hypotheses of the effects and functions of dreams.

1 Smith RC. A possible biologic role for dreaming. *Psychother Psychosom* 1984;**41**:167-76.
2 Nathan RJ, Rose-Itkoff C, Lord G. Dreams, first memories and brain atrophy in the elderly. *Hillside J Clin Psychiatry* 1981;**3**:139-48.
3 Smith RC. Do dreams reflect a biological state? *Journal of Nervous and Mental Diseases* 1987;**175**:201-7.
4 Haskell R. Dreaming, cognition and physical illness: part I. *Journal of Medical Humanities and Bioethics* 1985;**6**:46-56.
5 Miller L. On the neurophysiology of dreams. *Psychoanal Rev* 1989;**76**:375-401.
6 Shapiro CM, Catterall J, Montgomery I, Raab GM, Douglas NJ. Do asthmatics suffer bronchoconstriction during REM sleep? *BMJ* 1986;**292**:1161-5.
7 Shapiro CM, Douglas NJ. Psychophysiology of asthmatic patients at night. In: von Euler C, Katz-Solamon M, eds. *Respiratory psychophysiology*. Wenner-Gren International Symposium Series, vol 50. Basingstoke: Macmillan, 1988:53-62.

The portraits of Carl Gustav Jung and Sigmund Freud are Mary Evans Picture Library/Sigmund Freud copyright. The paintings by Moore, Burne-Jones, Botticelli, and Boucher are reproduced by permission of the Bridgeman Art Library.

PSYCHOTROPIC DRUGS AND SLEEP

Joel Eisen, James MacFarlane, Colin M Shapiro

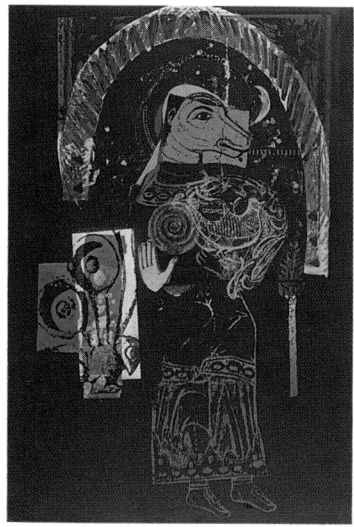

"Sula's dream" by Elspeth Lamb.

Factors in choosing the "right" drug

- Pharmacokinetics
- Side effects: benefits
- Side effects: disadvantages
- Contraindications
- Interaction with other drugs
- History of response
- Doctor's knowledge of drug

Our aim is to summarise how some of the most commonly used psychotropic drugs may affect sleep, and we will discuss them in three groups:

- Drugs used primarily to improve sleep
- Drugs used primarily to reduce sleepiness
- Drugs used primarily to treat particular psychiatric disorders which have secondary effects on sleep

It is important that before prescribing any treatment the doctor should try to make a precise diagnosis so that he or she can decide what kind of treatment is appropriate. For example, Mr Splitman, who complains of sleep disturbance during an acute exacerbation of schizophrenia, should be given treatment different from that given to Ms Downer, whose sleep disturbance is a feature of a major depressive episode. Mr and Mrs Kryer may benefit from psychotherapy for their recent bereavement, together with a drug to relieve secondary insomnia. Mr Bullneck's hypersomnolence, irritability, and mild depression could be a secondary feature of his sleep apnoea (diagnosed by overnight electrophysiological testing), and he will probably require treatment other than drugs. In contrast, young Phil Drowsey's performance at school is deteriorating, and he has withdrawn from most of his extracurricular social activities. This is, however, secondary to depressed alertness, not to depressed mood, despite apparently adequate nocturnal sleep, and suggests narcolepsy.

It is clear that drugs are only one of the treatments available for the various medicopsychiatric disorders, all of which have disturbed sleep as a common denominator. If drugs are indicated the doctor is often caught in a pharmaceutical "jungle"; choosing the right drug can be a formidable task, and the final selection depends on several factors.

Drugs used primarily to improve sleep

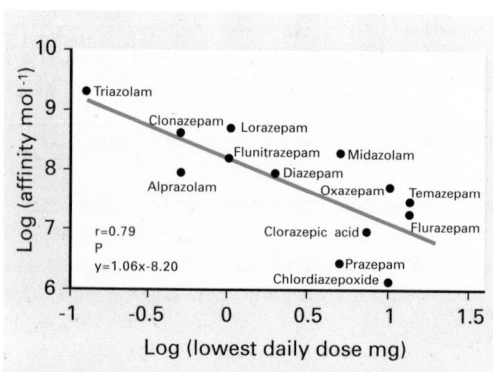

Benzodiazepine affinities in human brain and clinical dose.

Various hypnotic drugs that have been used in the past such as glutethimide, barbiturates, meprobamate, methaqualone, and methylprylone can be lethal; have great potential for misuse; and have no appreciable advantages over the newer compounds. For these reasons they have no place in modern treatment.

Hypnotic drugs are appropriate for the short term treatment (up to four weeks) of insomnia of recent onset caused by acute stress—for example, anxiety about examinations, or bereavement. Their use for chronic insomnia is more contentious, though they may be of benefit after the possibility of another sleep disorder has been ruled out and the causes of the insomnia have been properly investigated and treated.

Benzodiazepines have a characteristic influence on sleep architecture. They attenuate rapid eye movement (REM) and slow wave sleep, and increase stage 2 sleep. This may benefit patients whose problems are related to a particular stage of sleep such as dream anxiety attacks and night frights, but "REM rebound" occurs after treatment is discontinued, and patients may have an increase in the number of vivid or frightening dreams. In addition, tolerance to the hypnotic effects of the drugs is common after long term use.

Psychotropic drugs and sleep

Some newer hypnotic compounds (for example, zopiclone and zolpidem) seem to have similar sleep enhancing properties but are less likely to alter sleep architecture, and it is claimed that patients are much less likely to develop tolerance or dependence. Zopiclone may actually increase the amount of slow wave sleep, which is particularly relevant for those patients who complain of chronic fatigue or diffuse musculoskeletal discomfort, or both, and may be associated with reduction in both the quality and the quantity of slow wave sleep.

The onset of the hypnotic effect is regulated mainly by the drug's rate of absorption, but accumulation of the drug and its potential "carry over" effects and sedation during the day are related to the elimination half life of the drug and its active metabolites. For example, triazolam resulted in little accumulation and few daytime effects, but because of its short half life patients tended to have withdrawal effects between doses, which led to wakefulness in the early morning and rebound anxiety. In contrast, flurazepam, which has a long half life, may cause sedation during the day but has no rapid withdrawal effects.

These drugs are metabolised mainly in the liver and excreted in the urine. The dose does not have to be adjusted in patients with mild or moderate hepatic disease or renal failure, but in patients with severe liver disease a sedative that is not metabolised in the liver (such as oxazepam or lorazepam) is recommended. The sedative effects of benzodiazepines can be magnified in patients with coexisting brain disease and in elderly people, and they may require a reduced dose.

Pharmacokinetics of some hypnotic drugs

Pharmacokinetic characteristics	Drug	Mean (SD) $T_{1/2}$ (hours)	Dose (mg) Adult/elderly	Indications/comments
Slow absorption	Lorazepam	8	1·0-2·0/1·0	Sustains sleep; has residual daytime effects
	Oxazepam	8	15-30/10-20	Sustains sleep; has no residual effect; anxiolytic
Slow elimination	Flurazepam	64	15-30/15·0	Sustains sleep; has residual effects; anxiolytic
Slow elimination; pronounced distribution; rapid absorption	Diazepam	32	5-10/2·5-5·0	Sustains sleep; has residual effects; anxiolytic
Slow elimination; pronounced distribution	Nitrazepam	30	5·0/2·5-5·0	Sustains sleep; useful in the treatment of periodic movements
Intermediate elimination; pronounced distributution	Temazepam	8	10-60/10-20	Initiates sleep; has no residual effects
	Lormetazepam	9	1-2/0·5	Two formulations—one for sleep onset and one for maintenance
Rapid elimination	Zopiclone	5	3·75-7·5/3·75	Initiates sleep; no residual effects; no withdrawal effect
Extremely rapid elimination	Triazolam	3	0·125-0·25/0·125	Initiates sleep; has rebound insomnia and withdrawal effects.
	Zolpidem	2	10	Initiates sleep; has no residual effects; no withdrawal effects

Zopiclone and zolpidem are not benzodiazepines.

Drugs used primarily to reduce sleepiness

The class of drugs most widely prescribed to treat excessive sleepiness during the day are those that stimulate the central nervous system. Amphetamines were the first; they were unique in their pronounced alerting effect after a single oral dose, but the common side effects (which included irritability, tachycardia, and insomnia, as well as tolerance and dependence) made methylphenidate the preferred drug. It is more rapidly absorbed and has appreciably fewer sympathomimetic side effects. Pemoline, an oxazolidone derivative, is much less effective, but is tolerated well and has a longer half life. It is generally recommended for milder forms of sleepiness for which treatment with a stimulant is required—for example, narcolepsy. We have found that high doses of selegiline hydrochloride (up to 30 mg/day) are useful for both narcolepsy and nocturnal myoclonus.

All psychostimulants have profound effects on sleep. They reduce the total duration of sleep, REM sleep, and slow wave sleep, and increase the time taken to fall asleep and the fragmentation of sleep. These drugs must be given in the recommended divided doses, the highest being given in the morning and tapering to the last at 1600 or 1700 at the latest. For example, methylphenidate can be divided as follows: 20 mg in the morning, 10 mg at 1200, and 10 mg at 1600 (if necessary). To make sure that the treatment is appropriate, and that the optimal dosage regimen has been established, a "maintenance of wakefulness" test should be done before and after treatment to find out the degree of daytime sleepiness. The patient's sleep/wake routine must also be considered, as restriction of sleep is a common cause of hypersomnolence.

Pharmacological effects of some psychostimulant drugs

Drug	Alerting effect	Sympathomimetic effect	Dose (mg) Adult/elderly
Dexamphetamine	++++	++++	5-60/2·5-40
Methylphenidate	++++	+++	30-60/15-30
Pemoline	++	+	37·5-75/25-50

Commonly used preparations of methylphenidate and selegiline.

Psychotropic drugs and sleep
Drugs for psychiatric disorders with secondary effects on sleep

Pharmacological effects of antidepressant drugs

Drug	Sedative effect	Anticholinergic effect	Dose (mg) Adult/elderly
Tricyclic (tertiary amines):			
Amitriptyline	+++++	++++	150-200/100
Trimipramine	++++	+++	150-200/100
Doxepin	++++	+++	150-250/100
Imipramine	+++	+++++	150-200/100
Clomipramine	+++++	+++++	150-200/100
Tricyclic (secondary amines):			
Nortriptyline	++	+++	75-100/100
Protriptyline	+	+++	30-40/30
Desipramine	+	+	150-250/100
Tetracyclic:			
Maprotiline	++++	++	200-250/150
Mianserin	++++	+	30-90/30
Triazolopyridine:			
Trazodone	++++	++	100-25/100
Phenylpropylamine:			
Fluoxitine	+/−	+	20-40/10

Rate of insomnia and somnolence (%) associated with several newer antidepressants. Where a placebo was used for comparison the percentage is shown in parenthesis

Drug	Insomnia (v placebo)	Somnolence
Trazodone	6 (12)	41 (20)
Sertraline	16 (9)	13 (6)
Paroxetine	15	23
Fluoxetine	20 (7)	37 (15)
Fluvoxamine	11	26
Moclobemide	7 (5)	4 (6)
Buspirone	4 (2)	9 (10)

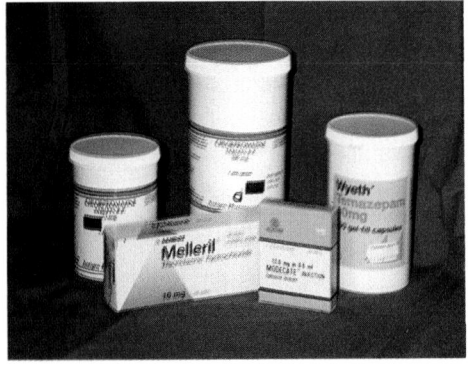

Some commonly used hypnotic and antipsychotic drugs.

Antidepressants

Tricyclic antidepressants and monoamine oxidase inhibitors have traditionally been used to treat depression. Recently their indications have been broadened to include panic disorders, agoraphobia, dysthymic disorders, depression in medical illness, and depression in schizophrenia.

Some antidepressant drugs have a mild alerting effect, which can be exploited in certain regimens of treatment. Mazindol, an imidazole derivative, is anorectic and has a mild stimulating effect on the central nervous system. Some other monoamine reuptake blockers such as protriptyline, voloxazine, fluoxetine, and some monoamine oxidase inhibitors, may actually improve alertness during the day, performance of psychomotor tasks, and cognitive functioning. Fluoxetine is a new antidepressant which has little if any anticholinergic activity and may increase anxiety. Surprisingly, formal sleep studies of this drug have not yet been published. Psychotropic drugs that have even mild activating effects should be taken early in the day to improve waking performance while minimising the possibility of iatrogenic insomnia.

The sedative effects of most of the cyclic antidepressants parallel their anticholinergic properties, so the tertiary amines are the most soporific and anticholinergic, and the secondary amines less so. Drugs such as amitriptyline and doxepin should be given later in the day, as agitated patients may benefit from their sedative side effects.

Antidepressant drugs cause immediate and profound effects on sleep architecture, of which pronounced suppression of REM sleep is the most important. This has been effectively exploited in non-psychiatric treatments so that symptoms associated with REM sleep, such as some apnoeas, and cataplexy in narcolepsy, may be brought under control. Clomipramine, which has the most suppressive effect on REM sleep, has been used in the treatment of recurrent severe nightmares. There are also increases in the amounts of slow wave and stage 1 sleep.

Antidepressant drugs should not be used purely as hypnotics. The choice of drugs to treat depression should take all other relevant factors into consideration, and the sedating effects of the drug should be particularly noted. There is an increasing practice of using an antidepressant combined with a hypnotic in the initial phase of treatment, particularly fluoxetine.

Monoamine oxidase inhibitors have a particular niche in the treatment of atypical depression, which is characterised by "reverse" neurovegetative symptoms such as hypersomnolence and hyperphagia.

Mood stabilising drugs

Lithium carbonate is the drug of choice for the prophylaxis of bipolar affective disorders. Less rigorously documented is its efficacy in the treatment of schizoaffective disorders, borderline personality disorders, and cyclothymic personality disorders. In the management of hypomania it is usually used in combination with a neuroleptic drug. It is also used alone for depression or to augment the antidepressant effect of one of the cyclic antidepressants. Studies of the effects of lithium on sleep have shown that it reduces the amount of REM sleep and postpones its onset. The amount of slow wave sleep increases in patients with mood disorders, and in some healthy controls. Hypomanic patients may become aware of a dulling of their alertness, but this may be partly the result of resolution of their illness. Some hypomanic patients dislike the restoration of a normal sleep/wake rhythm because they lose their sense of grandiose tirelessness. If frank sedation occurs when lithium is given, toxicity should be considered (>5 mmol/l).

Carbemazepine, which is similar in structure to the tricyclic antidepressant drugs, was first used in the 1960s to treat trigeminal neuralgia, but the indications for its use have been expanded to include various seizure disorders and the prophylaxis and acute treatment of bipolar affective disorders. Although its effects are comparable with those of lithium, its use as a mood stabiliser is reserved for patients who do not respond to lithium and, perhaps, for "rapid cyclers" (patients who have four or more episodes a year) because of rare reports of agranulocytosis and aplastic anaemia.

In healthy volunteers carbemazepine augments slow wave, and suppresses REM, sleep. Drowsiness is common at the start of treatment or when the dose is increased, but is nearly always transient.

Sodium valproate is usually used to treat epilepsy but is also useful in rapid cycling bipolar affective disorders that are refractory to other treatments such as lithium. It has fewer sedative side effects than carbemazepine, and sleep architecture is altered only slightly in healthy controls; the only appreciable long term effects are increases in the duration and depth of sleep, and a reduction in the time that it takes to get to sleep.

> Lithium, carbemazepine, and sodium valproate may all alter circadian rhythms

Some pharmacological properties of antipsychotic drugs

Clinical potency (least to most)	Sedation effects	Parkinsonian effects	Anticholinergic effects	Oral dose equivalent (mg)
Thioridazine	+ + + +	+	+ + + + +	100
Chlorpromazine	+ + + + +	+ +	+ + + +	100
Loxapine	+ + +	+ + +	+ +	10
Molindone	+	+ + +	+ +	10
Perphenazine	+ + +	+ + + +	+ +	10
Trifluoperazine	+	+ + + +	+ +	5
Thiothixene	+ +	+ + + +	+ +	5
Fluphenazine	+ +	+ + + + +	+ +	4
Haloperidol	+ +	+ + + + +	+	4

Conclusion

The cautious and considered use of hypnotic drugs (combined with behavioural modification) is an important part of the treatment of insomnia. The judicious use of stimulants in clearly diagnosed hypersomnolent patients is desirable.

Antipsychotic drugs

Antipsychotic drugs (or neuroleptics) are commonly used to treat schizophrenia as well as other psychotic conditions and delirium. They are also helpful as an adjunct to analgesic drugs in the relief of intractable pain because they induce a state of "psychic indifference." These drugs have comparable effects, but their side effects differ. In general the potent ones such as haloperidol are more likely to cause extrapyramidal symptoms such as dystonia, parkinsonism, and tardive dyskinesia, but are less likely to cause sedation, anticholinergic effects, and orthostatic hypertension. Some clinicians believe that paranoid patients become particularly distressed when they are sedated because they feel less in control, and these patients do best when given potent antipsychotic drugs.

These drugs do not have particular characteristic effects on sleep, but most tend to reduce periods of wakefulness and increase the duration of slow wave sleep when they are given in therapeutic doses. The amount of REM sleep can be increased or reduced, depending on the dose. There is a pronounced reduction in the duration of both REM sleep and overall sleep when the drugs are stopped.

We thank Dr Alan M Jackson for taking the photographs. "Sula's dream" by Elspeth Lamb is reproduced by permission of the artist. The figure of benzodiazepine affinities is based on data from Dr Elliott Richelson, Mayo Clinic, Jacksonville, and is reproduced with permission.

NON-PSYCHOTROPIC DRUGS AND SLEEP

Chris Idzikowski, Colin M Shapiro

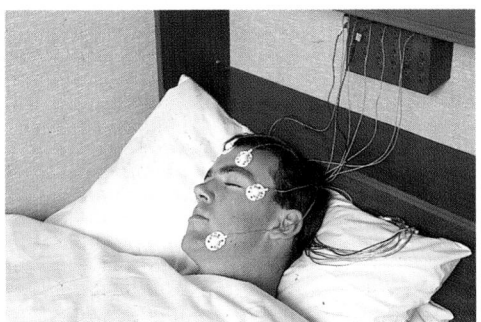

Assessment of sleep patterns.

Psychotropic drugs—drugs that affect the mental state—can also have peripheral effects. Similarly, drugs that are usually thought to have only peripheral actions may also influence the mental state, including affecting sleep patterns.

The mechanisms are varied. Some drugs penetrate the blood/brain barrier and directly affect the central nervous system (for example, antihistamines with sedative effects). Some drugs cause or aggravate conditions that disturb sleep—for example, sleep apnoea and restless legs. The effect may be extreme, as when sleep is broken by periods of wakefulness, or it may be subtle, as when only the electroencephalographic stages of sleep are disturbed.

General effects

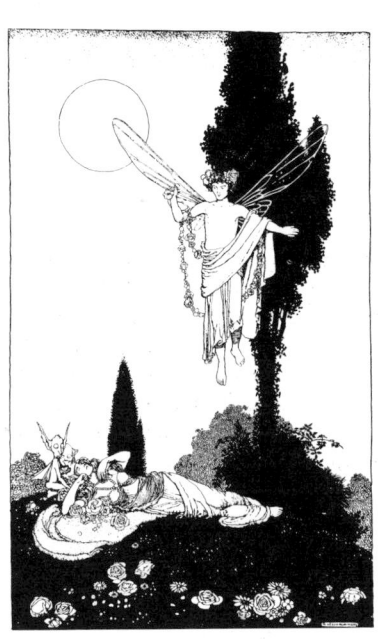

"A Midsummer Night's Dream" by W Heath Robinson.

The pharmacokinetic profile of any drug is important. Those with short half lives that are taken in the morning are unlikely to affect sleep the following night. It is also unlikely that they will accumulate (unless they have metabolites with long half lives) and affect sleep in that way. Those with long half lives that are given over long periods, however, will accumulate and produce high concentrations of the drug in the body.

To understand the effects of non-psychotropic drugs on sleep we must know:

● Whether the drug is likely to enter the central nervous system: its lipophilicity will indicate whether it will enter the brain, and so whether it will affect sleep.

● The receptor binding profile, which may predict the pharmacological action, particularly if it affects one of the main neurotransmitter systems (aminergic, cholinergic, or γ aminobutyric acid). Drugs that stimulate the noradrenergic system may disrupt sleep, and those that stimulate the cholinergic system may accelerate the onset of rapid eye movement (REM) sleep, and increase the amount of dreaming.

● Whether the drug has any peripheral effects that may impair ability to sleep. For example, drugs that cause or exacerbate the sleep apnoea/hypopnoea syndrome may disturb sleep (for example, benzodiazepines), but patients may not be aware of this and subsequently complain of daytime sleepiness. Drugs that alleviate pain may have the secondary effect of improving the quality of sleep.

When a patient presents with daytime sleepiness it may be either the direct effect of the drug, or a consequence of disturbed sleep at night.

Appetite suppressants

> Appetite suppressants cause both
> daytime sedation and disturbed sleep

Most appetite suppressants disturb sleep because they stimulate the central transmission of catecholamines. Amphetamine has the greatest effect but diethylpropion, mazindol, and phentermine also cause insomnia. Fenfluramine is the exception: it is chemically related to amphetamine, but its pharmacological action is primarily serotonergic. It releases serotonin from presynaptic sites and prevents it being taken up again; it causes both daytime sedation and disturbed sleep (by replacing sleep with periods of drowsiness and wakefulness); and it reduces the duration of REM sleep. It may increase the amount of slow wave sleep, but that may be as a consequence of disturbed sleep on the previous night.

Antiemetic drugs

Most antiemetic drugs penetrate the blood/brain barrier and probably sedate by their actions on the dopaminergic, histaminergic, or cholinergic neurotransmitter systems.

Hyoscine is a short acting, but powerful, central and peripheral antimuscarinic agent. It not only sedates, but also (by its action on the cholinergic system) reduces the amount of REM sleep and increases light (stage 2) sleep and body movements. REM sleep is increased on withdrawal of the drug.

Domperidone, which acts on the chemoreceptor trigger zone outside the blood/brain barrier, is a possible exception. Prochlorperazine, perphenazine, trifluorperazine, and thiethylperazine may all cause sedation.

> Most antiemetic drugs cause sedation. Domperidone is a possible exception

Antihistamines

Histamine is a neurotransmitter that plays a part in the regulation of sleep and wakefulness, so drugs that affect histamine transmission and enter the central nervous system will affect sleep. Many of the early antihistamines also had serotonergic, noradrenergic, and cholinergic activity and entered the central nervous system.

H_1 *antagonists*—The older antihistamines (such as triprolidine and promethazine) invariably caused daytime sleepiness. This has led to the development of drugs that do not cause sedation (such as astemizole, terfenadine, and loratadine); these drugs either do not penetrate the central nervous system, or enter it slowly, and they do not affect other neurotransmitter systems except in high doses. Cyproheptadine is a serotonin antagonist, and both increases the duration of slow wave sleep and reduces REM sleep.

H_2 *antagonists*—Cimetidine increases the duration of slow wave sleep, but ranitidine does not.

> New antihistamines have been developed that do not cause drowsiness
>
> *Examples*
> Astemizole
> Terfenadine
> Loratidine

Corticosteroids

The psychostimulant effects of glucocorticosteroids vary depending on the dose, the duration of treatment, and the reaction of the patient. Large doses can cause changes in behaviour and personality that range from nervousness, insomnia, euphoria, and mood swings to psychotic episodes that include both manic and depressive states, paranoia, and acute toxic psychoses. It is possible that these reactions are triggered by sleep disruption. The effects are most pronounced with dexamethasone and least with 6-methylprednisolone and prednylidene.

> Large doses of steroids can cause changes in behaviour and personality

Cardiovascular drugs

Antihypertensive drugs

α Methyldopa inhibits aromatic L-amino-decarboxylase, which plays a part in the synthesis of noradrenaline and serotonin. It increases the duration of REM sleep during the first half of the night at the same time as reducing the amount of slow wave sleep, and can cause both sedation and nightmares. Reserpine blocks the synthesis of amines in the brain and depletes stores of serotonin and catecholamines. It increases REM sleep and can cause depression, drowsiness, lethargy, and nightmares.

Adrenoceptor drugs

α *Agonists*—Clonidine is associated with insomnia and vivid dreams, particularly at the start of treatment, but in the laboratory it seems to suppress REM sleep and increase the duration of slow wave sleep. Children whose mothers were treated with clonidine during pregnancy have more disturbed sleep than those who were not.

> *Antihypertensive drugs* increase the duration of REM sleep
>
> *Clonidine* disturbs sleep patterns
>
> β *Blockers* have a varying effect on sleep, depending primarily on their lipophilicity—more water soluble drugs are less likely to enter the brain and have an effect on sleep

Non-psychotropic drugs and sleep

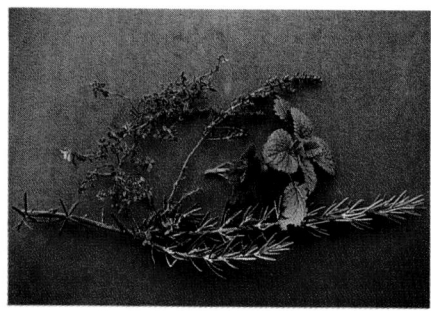

β Blocker		Partition coefficient
More water soluble		
Atenolol		0·02
Solatol		0·04
Nadolol	The more	0·07
Acebutolol	lipid soluble	0·7
Metoprolol	the drug the	1·0
Pindolol	more likely	0·8
Timolol	it is to cause	1·2
Oxprenolol	insomnia and	2·3
Labetalol	nightmares	11·5
Propranolol		20·2
More lipid soluble		

Partition coefficients of lipid solubilities of various β blockers. The more lipid soluble they are, the more likely to cause insomnia and nightmares.

α *Antagonists*—Indoramin and prazosin may both cause transient sedation at the start of treatment. Yohimbine increases the duration of REM sleep and reduces the duration of slow wave sleep; it is also alleged to have aphrodisiac properties, but there are no data to confirm this. It is not licensed in the United Kingdom.

β *Agonists*—Salbutamol (in a dose of 1·5 mg) has been investigated in a sleep laboratory but had no effect on sleep; pseudoephedrine on the other hand does disrupt sleep.

β *Antagonists*—The incidence of sleep disturbance depends primarily on the lipophilicity of the drug concerned, but partial agonist activity, membrane stabilisation, intrinsic sympathomimetic activity, stereospecificity, and affinity for other receptors may all affect the degree of sleep disturbance and daytime drowsiness. Propranolol, pindolol, and metoprolol all disturb sleep, though few effects have been noted with solatol. Acebutolol, alprenolol, atenolol, and oxprenolol all affect sleep, but simply switching from one β blocker to another may reduce the incidence of insomnia and increase compliance.

Propranolol blocks both β_1 and β_2 adrenoceptors; laboratory studies do not show any profound effects on sleep, though there is a reduction in the amount of REM sleep. It is, however, associated clinically with disturbed sleep and nightmares.

Diuretic drugs

Acetazolamide promotes a bicarbonate diuresis with consequent lowering of the pH value. It has been used prophylactically for acute mountain sickness and may be useful for central apnoea. Spironolactone may cause drowsiness. The timing of the dose of diuretic may cause disruption of sleep because of the need to pass urine during the night.

Hormones and vitamin A

> Sleep disturbances caused by hypothyroidism resolve when the condition is treated

Sex hormones—An unusual complication of androgens (and of anabolic steroids) is the obstructive sleep apnoea syndrome, particularly with nandrolone.

Human growth hormone—Most human growth hormone is released at night, so treatment with it is best given in the evening—the optimum point in the circadian cycle.

Thyroid hormones—Hypothyroidism is associated with little or no slow wave sleep and disturbed REM sleep. Sleep is restored to normal when the condition is treated.

Vitamin A—Acute poisoning with vitamin A (retinol) causes symptoms of drowsiness, sluggishness, irritability, and an irresistible desire to sleep.

Herbs

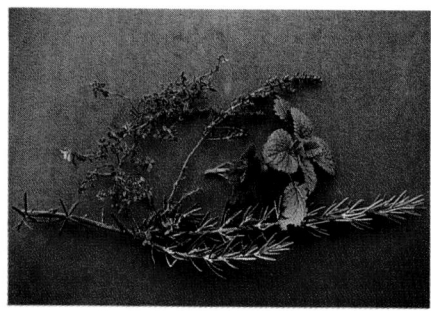

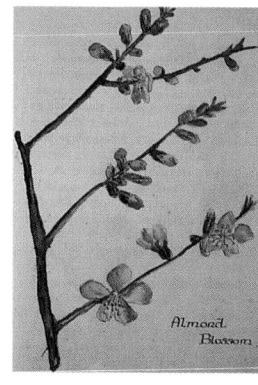

Almond Blossom

Almonds, camomile, catmint, fennel, ginseng, hops, indian hemp, lettuce, lime, marjoram, may blossom, melissa, mullein, oats, orange blossom, passion flower, poppy seed, rosemary, willow, and valerian are all traditionally thought to be sedatives. Most have not been investigated apart from heroin and the cannabinoids, but in some studies valerian has been found to improve the quality of sleep subjectively.

Herbs, including rosemary and camomile, that are believed to have sedative properties.

Conclusion

> Awareness of the effects of drugs on sleep may lead to more appropriate prescribing

Many drugs alter sleep architecture, which may alter compliance with the primary treatment, particularly if a drug (for example, fluoxetine) causes insomnia in a person with a condition (depression) in which disruption of sleep is poorly tolerated. In this example the side effect of the drug may perpetuate the primary illness. One option that is increasingly used is to give a hypnotic drug concurrently until the antidepressant has had an impact in decreasing insomnia associated with depression. If there is residual drug induced insomnia the hypnotic drug may be needed for the duration of drug treatment.

We thank Dr Alan M Jackson for taking the photographs of herbs. The previously unpublished watercolour of almond blossom was painted during the early 1920s and is reproduced with permission. "A Midsummer Night's Dream" is published by permission of the Mary Evans Picture Library.

RECREATIONAL DRUGS AND SLEEP

J R Stradling

Alcohol, nicotine, and caffeine are all powerful drugs that are commonly used during recreation. They all alter sleep (either initiation or maintenance), and in combination their effects can differ from their individual actions. Anyone who complains of poor sleep, therefore, should be asked how much of these drugs they consume. In many cases such people may have other causes for their insomnia—for example, anxiety or depression.

Trials of abstinence may need to last for several weeks before any benefit can be seen because of the length of time that any well established aberrant sleep pattern can take to improve.

> Alcohol, nicotine, and caffeine can all alter sleep, both separately and in combination

Smoking and nicotine

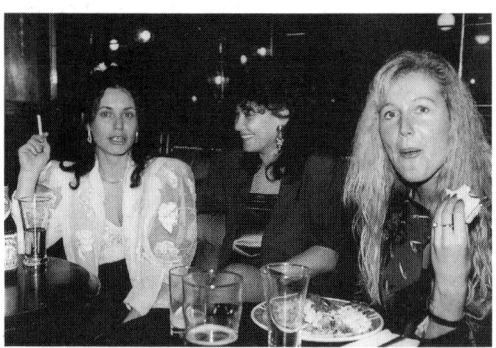

Smoking, drinking, and coffee can all adversely affect the quality of sleep.

Low blood concentrations of nicotine seem to cause mild sedation and relaxation and so a cigarette may promote sleep in an anxious person. As nicotine concentrations rise, however, the sedative effect is rapidly replaced by feelings of arousal and agitation: a cholinergic effect on nicotinic receptors. There is variation among subjects, and the half life of nicotine is about one to two hours. Smoking more than one cigarette within an hour of bedtime may therefore delay the onset of sleep, but insomnia later on in the night is unlikely to be caused by smoking during the evening. Heavy smokers certainly complain of sleeping less well than non-smokers, but there may be other important compounding variables. The average smoker sleeps about 30 minutes less than a non-smoker.

Nicotine withdrawal has mixed effects, and can produce both drowsiness and cortical arousal. This arousal produces the poor sleep that is often complained about by those who abruptly reduce a high cigarette consumption, but this persists only for two to four nights.

Alcohol

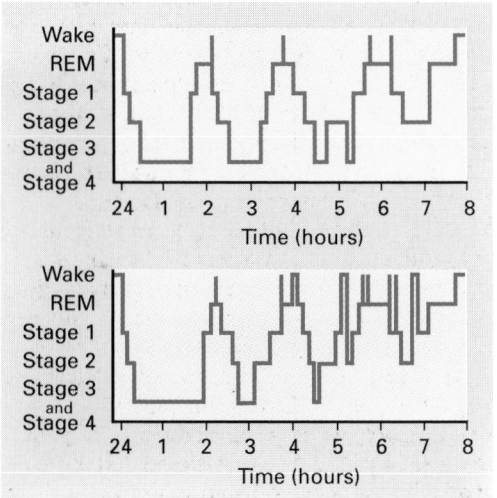

Hypnograms showing the effect of alcohol (bottom) on normal (top) sleep.

Alcohol is a brain sedative and promotes sleep. Its effects and those of many other sedatives are additive, and produce increases in slow wave sleep and a reduction in the amount of rapid eye movement (REM) sleep. Because it is metabolised fairly quickly the sedative effect declines as the night progresses. As with other short acting sedatives there is a rebound and arousal is heightened when blood alcohol concentrations fall to near zero; later in the night therefore there are an increased number of arousals (with increased catecholamine concentrations), as well as an increase in the amount of REM sleep. This may be quite pronounced in some people, who complain of recurrent awakening with tachycardia, sweating, headaches, and intense dream recall or nightmares. Though small doses of alcohol (one or two glasses of wine) are likely to promote sleep, more than this will produce increased arousal and insomnia later on in the night. Alcohol is metabolised at roughly one unit (a glass of wine or half a pint of beer) an hour, so after five drinks taken at about 2100 or 2200 the alcohol concentration will be near zero at 0300 and the sympathetic increase with more arousals will occur from this time onwards.

Soporific effect

Alcohol taken during the day will also reduce the arousal state and vigilance and promote sleep. The soporific effects of alcohol depend on the person's state of arousal before it was drunk. Alcohol taken in the morning after a good sleep, therefore, has a less soporific effect than that taken in the evening when the natural tendency to sleep is increasing. After sleep deprivation the effects of alcohol can be particularly devastating, with synergistic results on vigilance, so ability to drive after drinking alcohol will vary with the adequacy of the previous nights' sleep.

Snoring

In snorers the muscle relaxing properties of alcohol may further compromise the activity of the dilator muscles of the upper airway and allow complete collapse of the pharynx, which causes obstructive sleep apnoea. This will of course produce recurrent arousals, mainly early in the night, and such a person will then have an increased number of arousals both early and later on during the night. The ability of alcohol to cause or worsen snoring is known to many.

Alcohol misusers

Alcohol misusers often complain about sleep disturbances including hypersomnia, insomnia, and disruption of the sleep/wake cycle with frequent naps. The hypersomnia may be a direct result of taking alcohol, or can occur after a period of abstinence. Insomnia is more common, probably as a result of the mechanisms described above, as well as other specific medical problems such as gastritis. Sleep is fragmented during abstinence, and the amounts of both REM and slow wave sleep are reduced. These objective abnormalities, together with the subjective complaint of insomnia, may persist for several years after giving up alcohol and be one of the reasons for renewed drinking. There is some evidence that benzodiazepines will worsen rather than help these chronic symptoms. Treatment is difficult, but the usual advice for insomniac people is helpful: go to bed and wake up at regular times, do not take naps during the day, take regular exercise in the morning or afternoon, do not drink caffeine, and have a warm bath and a milky drink before going to bed.

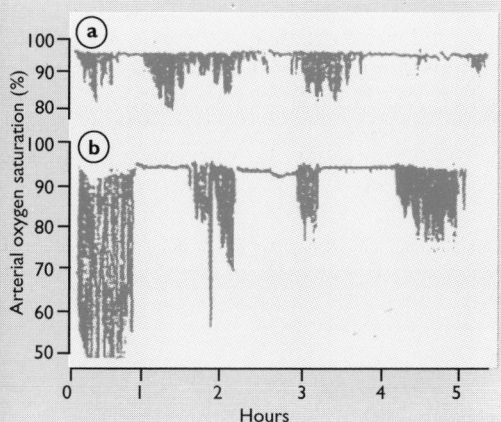

All night slow records of arterial oxyhaemoglobin saturation in a patient with obstructive apnoea (a) on a control night, and (b) after he had taken alcohol. On both nights the apnoea occurred only when he was supine.

Caffeine

Caffeine is an alerting chemical found in many drinks and some proprietary medicines that can be bought without prescription. Roasted ground coffee contains about 85 mg/150 ml cup, and strong brews many contain almost double this. Instant coffee has about 60 mg/140 g cup and decaffeinated coffee about 3 mg. Caffeine competes with adenosine (inhibitory neurotransmitter) receptors, causing cortical arousal. An intake of 300 mg clearly has an effect on sleep, with an increased number of arousals and reduced periods of REM sleep in most subjects tested; 500 mg causes the same degree of alertness as 5 mg of dexamphetamine. Though there is some variation among subjects, it is by no means as great as coffee drinkers claim. Even those who deny the effects of coffee on their sleep have an increased number of arousals after taking three cups of coffee near bedtime. Because caffeine has a long half life (five hours) it is not just the coffee that is consumed in the evening that is important. Drinking more than six cups of coffee a day is likely to cause an increased number of arousals and insomnia. Because two or three cups of coffee can be used to reduce the sleepiness during the day that follows minor sleep deprivation, a cycle may get established of poor sleep caused by ingestion of caffeine that is combated by the patient drinking yet more caffeine during the day.

Caffeine content (mg) of some common drinks (150 ml), chocolate (60 ml), and some drugs*

(one cup=150 ml, and one mug=200-230 ml)

	Range	Mean
Roasted and ground coffee (percolated)	64-124	83
Instant coffee	40-180	59
Decaffeinated coffee	2-5	3
Tea	8-91	27
Cocoa—African		6
Cocoa—South American		42
Ordinary cola drinks	12-19	15
Bar of milk chocolate		40
Migril (one tablet)		100
Cafergot (one tablet)		100
Antoin (maximum recommended daily dose		120
Doloxene compound (maximum recommended daily dose)		120
Cafadol, Solpadeine, Syndol (one tablet or capsule)		30
Hypon, Calpol Extra (one tablet or capsule)		10

*British National Formulary. London: BMA and Royal Pharmaceutical Society, 1992.

Recreational drugs and sleep
Alcohol and caffeine together

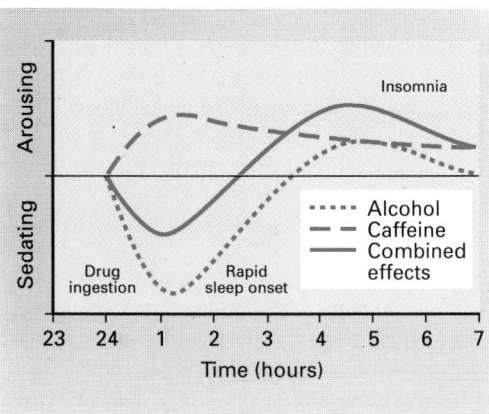

Combined effects of alcohol and caffeine on sleep.

Because of their opposing actions and different half lives, alcohol and caffeine taken together can produce particularly pronounced insomnia in the early hours of the morning. Alcohol's immediate sedative effect may reverse the alerting effects of caffeine. By about 0300 or 0400 the alcohol will have been metabolised; this will cause a rebound increase in cortical arousal that will now add to the alerting effects of the caffeine, which is only half metabolised by this time.

The photograph is reproduced with permission of Ulrike Preuss.

The table of caffeine contents has been adapted from Dews PB, ed. *Caffeine*. Berlin:Springer, 1984:61, and the records of oxyhaemoglobin saturation are reproduced from Issa FG, Sullivan CE. Alcohol, snoring and sleep apnoea. *J Neurol Neurosurg Psychiatry* 1982;**45**:353-9, with permission.

ILLICIT DRUGS AND SLEEP

L W Reinish, P Sandor, Colin M Shapiro

> **Cross tolerance of the effects on sleep of various misused substances**
>
> **Narcotics:**
> All other narcotics (codeine, heroin, pethidine, methadone, morphine)
>
> **Ethyl alcohol:**
> Benzodiazepines, barbiturates, meprobamate, glutethimide, methaqualone
>
> **Benzodiazepines:**
> Barbiturates, ethyl alcohol, carbamazepine
>
> **Barbiturates:**
> Glutethimide, benzodiazepines (though these may not prevent seizures during barbiturate withdrawal), meprobamate, ethyl alcohol, methaqualone
>
> **Hallucinogens**
> Other hallucinogens, lysergic acid diethylamide, psilocybin, mescaline (though tetrahydrocannabinol may induce relaxation and sleep)
>
> **Stimulants**
> Other stimulants (dexamphetamine, methylphenidate, fenfluramine) but not cocaine

Misusers of drugs commonly complain of sleep disruption, but there are few publications about it. Patients may misuse drugs ostensibly for their effects on sleep (for example, alcohol and marijuana), but both these drugs can cause insomnia under certain circumstances. Many former drug misusers continue to have problems with sleep for up to a year after they have given up drugs. Family doctors who treat such patients face the dilemma of whether they should prescribe benzodiazepines to such patients; unfortunately the alternative is often that the patient reverts to using illicit drugs.

There are certain terms associated with the misuse of drugs:

Tolerance is a sign of physical adaptation to commonly used substances, but it does not develop to all the effects of a given drug at the same speed. For example, tolerance to the sedating effects of barbiturates develops quickly, but not to their anticonvulsant or respiratory depressing effects.

Cross tolerance is the development of tolerance to another drug in the same or a similar class.

Patients become *physically dependent* when tolerance develops and there are physiological disturbances if the drug is withdrawn, and they become *psychologically dependent* when they use the drug to provide relief from disturbing symptoms such as anxiety or pain, and when they fear the consequence of not using the drug.

During *withdrawal* the signs and symptoms that present tend to be the opposite of the usual effects of the drug. Short acting substances that act rapidly are more likely to produce tolerance and dependence than the longer acting equivalents, and are usually associated with more severe withdrawal symptoms.

Cannabinoids

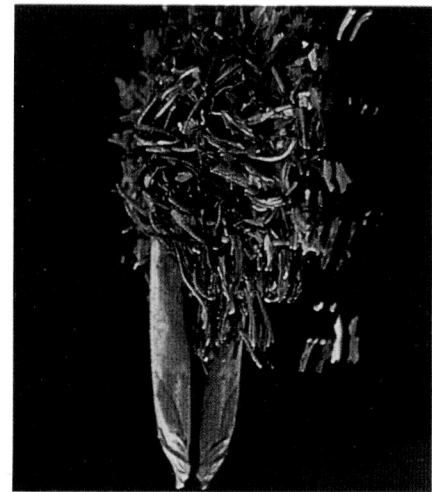

"Manicured" or harvested marijuana.

δ^9-Tetrahydrocannabinol is the active hallucinogen of marijuana, which is prepared from the flowering top and leaves of the plant *Cannabis sativa*. The average content of a marijuana cigarette is 2·5-5·0 mg (between 1% and 2% by weight). Hashish is derived from a dried and concentrated exudate of the flowers and contains several times more of the active drug. Marijuana is usually smoked, and about 50% of the total dose is absorbed into the bloodstream. The subjective effect usually peaks within about 30 minutes, and disappears within three hours. If it is taken orally the bioavailability is about a third of that when it is smoked, the subjective effect starts about 45 minutes later, and it persists for up to five hours. It is metabolised in the liver and taken up by fatty tissue.

Marijuana reduces the amount of rapid eye movement (REM) sleep and initially increases slow wave sleep, but the latter effect is reversed after several days' use. The effect is potentiated by alcohol. It is a mild anxiolytic, which helps to induce sleep. Habitual heavy users develop a syndrome that is characterised by lassitude, poor judgment, and excessive sleep, and regular use produces tolerance and mild physical dependence. Abrupt withdrawal is associated with sleep disturbances, anxiety, sweating, and loss of appetite.

A study of the effects of the antenatal use of marijuana on babies' sleep showed that sleep was disturbed in those babies whose mothers had taken marijuana; they spend more time awake and less time in the deeper stages of sleep, and had more frequent body movements. The authors suggested that marijuana affects the maturation of various neuronal systems that have a role in initiation or maintenance of sleep and wakefulness.

Illicit drugs and sleep
Narcotic analgesics

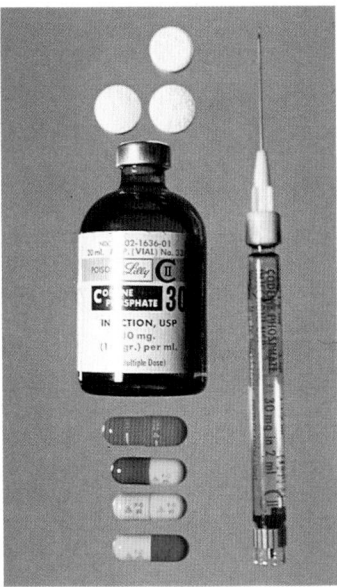

Synthetic narcotics.

Narcotic analgesics can be natural (morphine and codeine), semisynthetic (heroin), or synthetic (methadone and pethidine). The naturally occurring ones are made from refined opium, which is a tar like exudate of the pods of the poppy *Papaver somniferum*. Morphine and heroin are often taken by intravenous or subcutaneous injection, because if they are taken orally the amount absorbed from the "first pass" effect of liver metabolism is greatly reduced. The oral preparations are, however, popular among some drug misusers because they are easier to obtain and the quality is more consistent. The drugs can also be inhaled or smoked. Tolerance develops quickly with regular use.

Intravenous injection of narcotic analgesics produces a pleasurable rush, which facilitates addiction. After the rush the user enters a dreamlike, mildly drowsy state which is called the "nod" because of the nodding motions of the head that often occur. The effects on sleep are dose related and include delayed onset, fragmentation, increased periods of wakefulness, increased muscle tone and reductions in slow wave and REM sleep. Heroin is about twice as potent as morphine in producing these effects, and tolerance to them develops with regular use. In extremely high doses narcotics can cause sedation that may progress to coma.

Withdrawal

Sudden withdrawal produces a typical pattern of sleep changes; about eight to 12 hours after the last dose the user experiences an agitated sleep called the "yen", which may last for several hours. The withdrawal symptoms reach maximum intensity after 36-72 hours, and include increasing irritability and a pattern of sleep disruption similar to "morphine insomnia." Many narcotic misusers also misuse other drugs including barbiturates and benzodiazepines in an effort to achieve the sedative effect of the narcotic to which they have become tolerant, so complications may be related to withdrawal of other substances. The insomnia that occurs during withdrawal of narcotics may become persistent and be accompanied by depression and anxiety in those who continue to abstain.

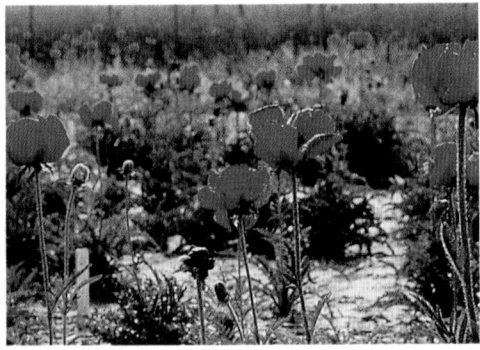

Field of poppies.

Treatment of narcotic withdrawal

Withdrawal, also called detoxification, is usually treated by substitution of methadone, initially 10-20 mg orally. This should suppress withdrawal symptoms within 30-60 minutes, but if necessary a further 5-10 mg may be given. A dose of 10-20 mg may be given after 12 hours if necessary. The total dose should be repeated the next day, the total daily dose not exceeding 40 mg. In hospital the methadone should then be withdrawn over the next five to 10 days by reducing the daily dose by 5 mg/day. Outpatient detoxification may take up to three weeks. Clonidine has been used instead of methadone but is less well established and can cause hypotension and rebound hypertension when it is discontinued. Babies born to mothers who are dependent on narcotics experience acute withdrawal symptoms including restlessness, crying, irritability, and rhinorrhoea, which may persist for several weeks or months.

Cocaine

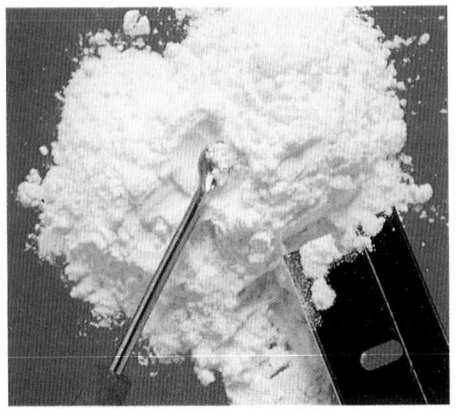

Cocaine hydrochloride.

Cocaine is a central nervous system stimulant with euphoric and alerting effects which is obtained from the leaves of the tree *Erythroxylon coca* that grows in Peru and Bolivia. It suppresses the appetite and the need for sleep. It may be inhaled or injected, and its effects start to decrease after 30-40 minutes. Tolerance has not been shown in humans. Cocaine hydrochloride (the product of refining cocaine from the *Erythroxylon coca* tree) cannot be smoked as it decomposes when it is heated. "Crack" cocaine is the free base form of cocaine, which melts at 90°C. Crack cocaine is sold in a potent form, but may contain adulterants such as lignocaine or amphetamines.

The effects on sleep are similar to those of other psychostimulants, and include delayed onset and reduced REM and slow wave sleep. People who use the drug regularly are commonly in a state of chronic sleep deprivation. Abrupt withdrawal results in depression and long periods of sleep with increased REM activity, which are probably a rebound effect from the previous sleep deprivation. Their severity is related to the duration of misuse and the dose. Desipramine may be helpful in reducing the craving and helping the patient to abstain.

Cocaine free base   Cocaine hydrochloride

cid base reactions of cocaine.

allucinogens

> Hallucinogens do not have a direct effect on sleep but may cause psychiatric disturbances

anabolic steroids

> Discontinuation can cause sleep disturbance

Psychostimulants and appetite suppressants

> - Amphetamines cause a reduction in REM and slow wave sleep
> - Fenfluramine is not associated with changes in REM sleep
> - "Ecstasy" totally suppresses REM sleep

Benzodiazepine misuse

> Prescribing practices for benzodiazepines have been re-evaluated

Illicit drugs and sleep

Infants exposed to cocaine in utero are at increased risk of neurological abnormalities including perinatal cerebral infarction, intracranial haemorrhage seizures, and disturbed behaviour. An electroencephalographic study of such infants showed that nearly 6% showed a discordance between the clinical and electroencephalographic sleep state, compared with normal infants. Affected infants also began mature, continuous slow wave sleep at a significantly younger age than the controls.

Hallucinogens are structurally similar, though they can be naturally occurring (psilocybin, dimethyltryptamine, mescaline), semisynthetic (d-lysergic acid diethylamide—LSD), and synthetic (phencyclidine, 3,4-methylenedioxyamphetamine, ketamine). They can all be synthesised in the laboratory.

They do not have a direct effect on sleep and there is no reported withdrawal syndrome, but people who take large doses may experience "bad trips" that lead to an agitated psychosis and disruption of normal sleep, and can last for a day or two. Phencyclidine is associated with a psychotic syndrome which can last for about five days and causes paranoid psychosis, anorexia, irritability, unpredictable aggressive behaviour, and insomnia.

Drugs such as stanozolol have been used by athletes to improve performance and physique. Discontinuation can cause depression and both insomnia and hypersomnia.

Amphetamines (such as dexamphetamine and methylphenidate) increase wakefulness and cause insomnia, and electroencephalographic changes during sleep while the drugs are being taken include appreciable reductions in both REM and slow wave sleep. Taken over a long period the drugs can cause tolerance to their effects on both alertness and sleep. Abrupt withdrawal is associated with lethargy, depression, and a rebound increase in REM sleep. When high doses of amphetamines are taken intermittently by drug misusers these withdrawal symptoms are referred to as "crashing." If there is still a mood disorder after a period of two to four weeks of withdrawal it should be investigated, and treated if indicated.

Fenfluramine is structurally related to the amphetamines and is used to treat obesity. Unlike the other amphetamines, therapeutic doses of fenfluramine (60-120 mg daily) typically cause drowsiness and are not associated with changes in REM sleep. There is subjective evidence that high doses (60 mg/day) of dexfenfluramine, the dextrorotatory isomer of fenfluramine, impair the quality of sleep.

Methylenedioxymethamphetamine, commonly known as "ecstasy," is a misused drug that is structurally related to amphetamine. It produces a combination of stimulant (similar to amphetamine) and hallucinogenic effects in humans. "*Eve*," 3,4-methylenedioxyethamphetamine, produces psychotropic effects similar to those produced by ecstasy. Sleep studies in healthy volunteers showed that after a single dose of eve 140 mg the subjects fell asleep normally but awoke 30-90 minutes later. After they had gone back to sleep REM sleep was totally suppressed for the remainder of the night. These changes are similar to those caused by other amphetamines.

Benzodiazepines are commonly misused either alone or in combination with other drugs not for their hypnotic properties, but for their sedative and anxiolytic effects and to relieve the side effects of other drugs. This misuse has prompted the regulatory bodies and the manufacturers to respond, and prescribing practices have been re-evaluated. For example, the misuse of the intravenous preparation of temazepam resulted in an "abuse resistant" gel formulation. Temazepam is nearly insoluble in water and forms a precipitate, so those misusers who dissolve the gel in water to inject it intra-arterially may develop microemboli that are initiated by the precipitate. Attempts to limit the misuse of benzodiazepines by changing their formulation may therefore be of limited usefulness.

Illicit drugs and sleep
Conclusions

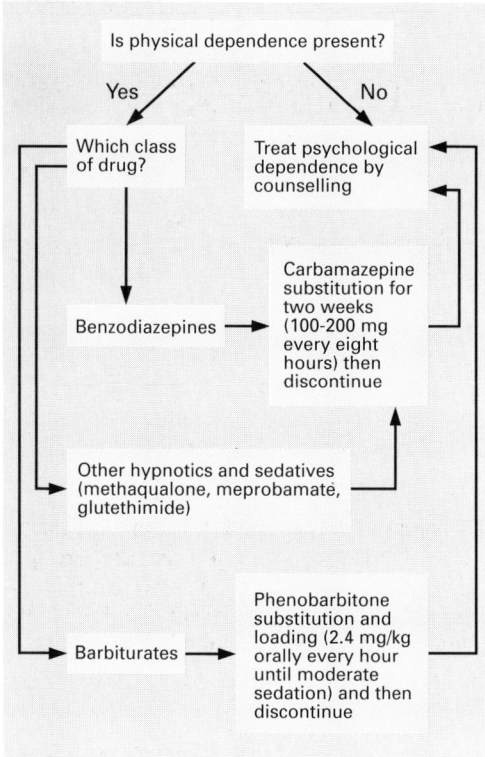

Algorithm showing treatment of withdrawal from hypnotics and sedatives.

Though the effects of specific drugs on sleep are important, there is evidence that there are also individual personal factors that affect the severity of withdrawal symptoms—that is, some patients may be significantly more prone to sleep disruption during withdrawal of any drug than others.

Many people have disrupted sleep as a result of misuse of illicit drugs, excessive use of recreational drugs, and taking "over the counter" products that purport to improve sleep. These drugs may not only effect the sleep of the user, but can have an impact on others such as the newborn babies of mothers who misuse drugs.

WITHDRAWAL FROM HYPNOTIC DRUGS

Peter Tyrer

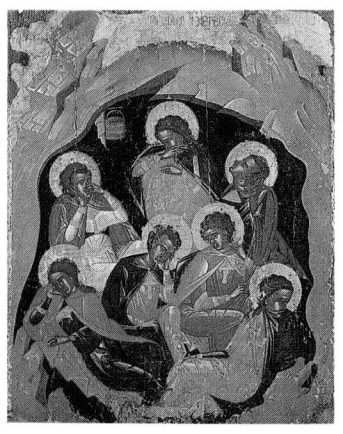

The seven sleepers of Ephesus were Christian soldiers who were emtombed in a cave while escaping religious persecution during the third century. They slept until the reign of Theodosius II (408-50) who, on hearing of their miraculous experience, was converted to Christianity.

As well as the traditional sedative/hypnotic group of drugs that relieve anxiety by day and promote sleep at night there are several other groups of drugs that are used to treat insomnia—particularly antidepressant, antipsychotic, and antihistamine drugs. As they differ substantially in their pharmacological and clinical effects on withdrawal I will consider them separately.

Sedative/hypnotic drugs

The main drugs in this group are benzodiazepines, but chloral derivatives (for example, chloral hydrate, triclofos, and dichloralphenazone), chlormezanone, and chlormethiazole are also used. Barbiturates and similar drugs (for example, glutethimide, methyprylone, and meprobamate) now have no place in the treatment of insomnia (see article on psychotropic drugs). Alcohol may also be included in this group. All these drugs act by facilitating transmission of the inhibitory neurotransmitter, γ-aminobutyric acid (GABA) in the central nervous system. When problems arise during withdrawal they can be regarded mainly as symptoms of GABA deficiency. Many hypnotic drugs suppress the rapid eye movement (REM) phase of sleep and there is a compensatory excess after withdrawal. This adds to the sleep disturbance.

Nature and incidence of withdrawal problems

The main problem after withdrawal from sedative/hypnotic drugs is a temporary increase in the severity of insomnia within seven days of stopping treatment. This normally lasts for one to three weeks (but can last up to two months) before it returns to prewithdrawal levels, and it is commonly termed "rebound insomnia." This is an appropriate term if the insomnia is not as pronounced as it was before the treatment started, but is better described as "recoil" or "overshoot" insomnia if it is severe and leads to fewer hours of sleep than before the drug was taken.

Predicting dependence on hypnotic drugs	
Factor	*Score*
Benzodiazepine	3
High mean dose*	2
Duration of treatment more than 3 months	2
Dependent personality (or previous dependence on drugs or alcohol)	2
Short elimination half life (<8 h)	2
Evidence of tolerance or escalation of dosage	.2
Total	

*Dose higher than mean of range given in *British National Formulary*

Score

0	No dependence, abrupt withdrawal appropriate
1-4	Some risk of dependence, gradual withdrawal over two weeks
5-8	Strong risk of dependence, gradual withdrawal over 4-12 weeks
8-13	Dependence almost certainly present, gradual reduction associated with formal withdrawal programme

Withdrawal from hypnotic drugs

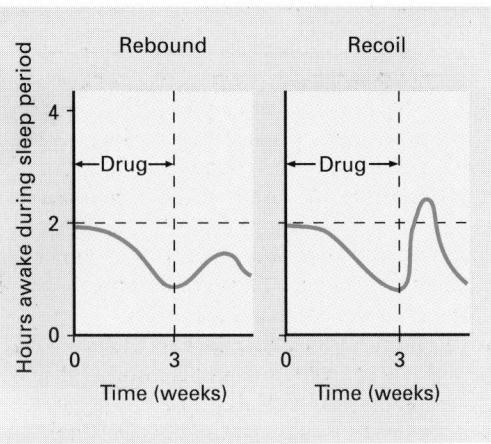

Rebound and recoil insomnia.

In addition to further insomnia, patients also experience other symptoms during the day including anxiety and its bodily manifestations (tremor, palpitations, dizziness, muscular tension, and pains); and perceptual distortions of noise (hyperacusis and tinnitus), touch (hyperaesthesiae, itching, and tingling sensations), and movement. Epileptic seizures, psychotic phenomena, and confusion may occur within seven days of withdrawal, but are rare.

Differences between drugs

The time and severity of rebound insomnia depend largely on the rate of metabolism and excretion of the drug. The elimination half life (the time taken for 50% of the drug to be inactivated) is a useful index of these differences. In general, the withdrawal symptoms after a drug with a short half life has been stopped occur sooner, are more severe, but last for a shorter time than the equivalent symptoms with drugs that have longer half lives. It is claimed that newer hypnotic drugs such as the cyclopyrrolones (for example, zopiclone) do not have associated rebound insomnia. Those that are available have intermediate half lives. One strategy for withdrawing a patient from long term hypnotic use is to switch to an alternative class of hypnotic drug—for example, from a benzodiazepine to a cyclopyrrolone. A four week course of the new drug should be given and then hypnotic treatment (in a patient primed to expect it) stopped.

Benzodiazepines grouped according to their elimination half lives			
Very short half life (up to 4 h)	Short half life (4-12 h)	Intermediate half life (12-20 h)	Long half life (>20 h)
Triazolam* Loprazolam*	Lormetazepam* Temazepam* Zopiclone***	Lorazepam Oxazepam	Nitrazepam* Flurazepam* Diazepam** Chlordiazepoxide*

*Drugs used primarily as hypnotics
**Drugs with short half lives that have active metabolites with long half lives and which are therefore long-acting when given over a long period
***Non-benzodiazepine with some characteristics different from other benzodiazepine hypnotics

Other sedative/hypnotic drugs

Other drugs in this group are similar to benzodiazepines with regard to withdrawal symptoms except that factors other than half life are more important in withdrawal. Barbiturates, alcohol, methyprylone, and glutethimide are associated with more tolerance and escalation of dose as well as with withdrawal reactions; chlormethiazole has many similarities to the benzodiazepines; and chloral hydrate derivatives give fewer problems after withdrawal than others in this group, but are less efficacious.

> Chloral hydrate derivatives cause fewer problems, but are less effective, than other drugs

Antidepressant and antihistamine drugs

> Antidepressants can cause rebound panic on occasions if they are withdrawn abruptly

Antidepressant drugs are often prescribed for patients who cannot sleep, not least because it is common for depressed patients to have insomnia. These drugs help insomnia in two ways—by their immediate sedative actions (most pronounced with the tricyclic antidepressants such as amitriptyline, trimipramine, and dothiepin), and by relieving both anxiety and depression after regular doses for several weeks. Antihistamines are also sedative (and indeed the sedative effects of antidepressant drugs are partly a result of their antihistaminic effects). If withdrawal of antidepressants is abrupt (particularly if the patient has been taking a large dose) symptoms of severe anxiety, including panic, are possible. These can usually be avoided by gradual reduction of the dose over four weeks.

Antipsychotic drugs

> Antipsychotic drugs rarely cause dependence and may be chosen as hypnotics in patients prone to dependence

Though in high doses antipsychotic drugs are used primarily for the treatment of schizophrenia and affective psychoses, they have sedative actions in low doses (for example, chlorpromazine 50 mg/day). Drugs with greater anticholinergic action (for example, thioridazine) are more sedative than those which act mainly on dopamine receptors (for example, flupenthixol). The main advantage of the anticholinergic type of drugs is that they are not prone to cause dependence and so withdrawal seldom causes any problems. Long term treatment is not advisable because of the risk (albeit low at these doses) of tardive dyskinesia.

Preventing and reducing withdrawal symptoms

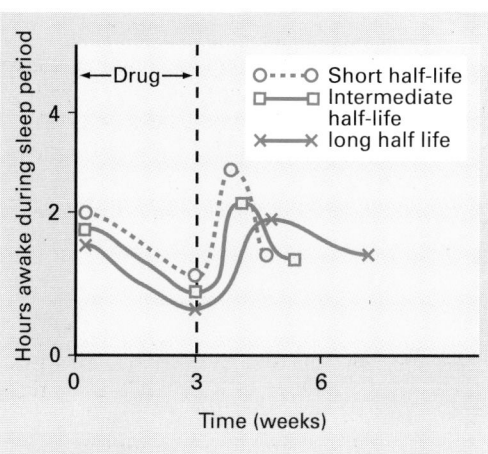

Differences in timing and intensity of withdrawal symptoms with benzodiazepines.

New symptoms can arise during withdrawal

Often the first evidence of dependence on hypnotic drugs is noticed during withdrawal. As dependence, once established, is difficult to treat, it is better to anticipate problems of withdrawal wherever possible. By assessing the various factors that contribute to dependence, both the duration of drug treatment and the mode of withdrawal can be selected to minimise symptoms.

Most of the factors that contribute to dependence have already been discussed. In general, the greater the amount of drug taken and the more rapidly it is withdrawn the greater the risk of dependence.

The influence of personality is also important. Patients with dependent personalities rely to a large extent on external forms of support including people and drugs, and when this support is withdrawn they have great difficulty in adjustment. Such patients often rely a great deal on their medical attendants (particularly their general practitioners) for such support and are sometimes described as "fat folder" patients because of the impressive width of their medical records. It is sometimes (accurately) said that the single most important factor in withdrawing a patient from dependency on hypnotic drugs is the relationship between the patient and the doctor.

Though rebound phenomena are neurophysiologically universal, certain patients are more prone to develop greater dependence on hypnotic drugs. Only about 30% to 40% of patients experience clinical problems in the form of withdrawal symptoms. New symptoms can also arise after a drug has been stopped, which are unrelated to its pharmacological actions ("pseudowithdrawal" symptoms). This is an example of the nocebo effect (nocebo=I will harm), the converse of the placebo effect. As public awareness of problems of withdrawal after taking tranquillising and hypnotic drugs increases, the nocebo effect assumes greater importance and complicates the interpretation of withdrawal symptoms.

Withdrawal programmes

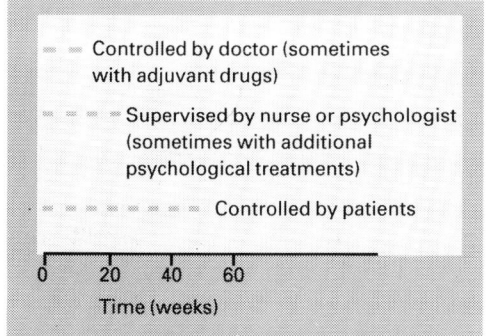

Types of withdrawal programme in patients dependent on hypnotic benzodiazepines

The simplest form of withdrawal programme is gradual withdrawal over a period varying from two weeks to many months. This permits adaptive changes to take place in the central nervous system that reduce the perturbation of withdrawal. The reduction can be supervised by the clinician or in some cases left primarily to the patient (though monitored medically through review of prescriptions). If reduction is planned over a long period (for example, six to 12 months) it is preferable for the patient to take the main role in planning the programme unless there is additional help from other therapists, including psychologists, community nurses, psychiatrists, and self help organisations. Formal withdrawal programmes can include yoga, meditation, hypnotherapy, and cognitive therapy; these non-pharmacological treatments of insomnia can help to counteract the severity of withdrawal symptoms as well as promoting sleep in their own right.

"Postwithdrawal" syndrome

Main features of postwithdrawal syndrome

- Persistence of insomnia more than eight weeks after complete withdrawal
- Greater vulnerability to stress
- Anxiety and irritability during the day
- Temporary resolution with benzodiazepines

Although rebound and recoil insomnia last for a period of only one to three weeks, problems often continue after this time. These cannot be described easily in the language of pharmacological dependence, because they can last for up to nine months after withdrawal. There is evidence that this "postwithdrawal" syndrome is the result of a delay in neurophysiological adjustment after withdrawal of a drug, during which there is reappraisal of the perception of threat. In other words, the patient has to relearn how to cope with stress and is unsettled while this is taking place.

If insomnia persists after this period both clinician and patient are faced with a difficult decision. If drug treatment is reinstituted it is likely to be long term or permanent. While this option is not attractive it may be the only realistic one in some cases, and can be chosen when the benefits achieved are greater than the consequences of dependence.

The illustration of the seven sleepers of Ephesus is from Greek Ministry of Culture. *From Byzantium to El Greco: Greek frescoes and icons.* Athens: Byzantium Museum of Athens, 1987.

LEGAL ASPECTS OF SLEEP AND ALERTNESS

R A A McCall Smith, Colin M Shapiro, A Moscovitch

Medicolegal aspects of alertness

Driving
Occupational
Social
- Liability of individual
- Liability of health care provider
- Duty to notify regulating authorities
- Industrial obligations (regarding) timing of work

Sleep related violence

Parasomnias
Behavioural disorder during REM sleep

Effects of medications on alertness and performance

Recognition and treatment of sleep conditions

Role of the sleep laboratory in assessing sleep related function

---

Sleep disorders and lack of alertness can cause various legal problems, and the association between daytime sleepiness and accidents is well known. Injuries to other people may result in insurance claims and injuries to the patient may result in claims against the doctor. In the United States there are roughly 200 000 sleep related motor vehicle accidents each year; they are the result not of delayed reaction times but of diminished vigilance and they occur when traffic is light. Disproportionately large numbers of sleep related accidents involve only one vehicle, and are fatal.

Several facets of criminal law relate to sleep disorders. Violence during sleep is rare, but its consequences may be grave. It is a vexing question whether a person who causes harm while sleepwalking is criminally liable. An outline of these issues is given in the box.

The doctor's civil liability for a patient's lack of alertness

---

Case settled by Medical Defence Union 1990

An 18 year old boy consulted his family doctor because he had had a blackout. The doctor arranged for the boy to have an electroencephalogram, and advised him not to drive in the meantime. The doctor discussed the results of the examination with the physician who had carried it out and, though no full report was given, the doctor formed the impression that it did not show signs of epilepsy.

The doctor therefore advised the patient that he could drive, and three weeks later the boy had a seizure while driving his car and caused serious injury to his passenger. The passenger sued the driver, who in turn sued the doctor for negligence in that he failed to advise him correctly about the risk entailed in driving. The case was settled for a substantial amount of money.

When a doctor should warn a patient

In a case dealt with by the Medical Defence Union in 1989, a family doctor failed to warn a patient about the risk of driving when taking diazepam (which had been prescribed) at the same time as alcohol. The insurers admitted that the doctor had a duty to issue a warning, though in the case in question the cause of the damage was far from clear because the patient was misusing other drugs at the same time.

The so called "Bolam standard" (named after the Bolam case in 1954) specifies that a doctor must practise with the ordinary skill of a competent practitioner, and provides that a course of action will not be negligent if it meets the approval of a responsible body of opinion within the profession. This standard applies to all forms of treatment and diagnosis.

Failure to take the possibility of a sleep disorder into account could, in some cases, amount to negligence on the part of a general practitioner. In most circumstances the patient who experiences daytime sleepiness will be aware of the fact and will be expected to take his own precautions against the possibility of injury. An insomniac patient who tends to fall asleep at the wheel of his car when driving during the day is the author of his own misfortune, and can hardly claim that his doctor should have warned him against driving when sleepy. There may be liability, however, when there is something unusual about the patient's lack of alertness and when he may not necessarily be expected to know what risk he is running by engaging in a particular activity. An example of this is a case settled by the Medical Defence Union in 1990.

It is becoming increasingly apparent that the impact of various drugs, including sedative antidepressants, tranquillisers, and some hypnotics, cause more daytime sedation than alcohol in terms of reduced psychomotor performance, thereby seriously affecting a person's ability to drive or operate machinery competently. This raises a potentially awkward problem for doctors who, though they acknowledge both the importance of alertness and the legal hazards involved in carrying out demanding or complex tasks (such as driving) while unfit, may still be reluctant to do anything that might discourage patients from complying with treatment. This is compounded by the fact that the interactions of many drugs that may affect alertness are not fully appreciated. Some of these interactions may not be anticipated — for example, some forms of insulin may interact with simple benzodiazepine hypnotics by differentially altering liver metabolism. It may therefore be difficult to predict the chance of a particular patient causing harm as a result of reduced alertness. Caution suggests that the doctor should warn the patient of the possibility.

vil liability of the patient

> Driving instruction manuals provide information about the use of alcohol but not about alertness

> Tell patients to open the windows of the car, play loud music, eat an apple, or have a caffeinated drink if they feel sleepy while driving. These will help only briefly, however, and **the best solution is to pull off the road and have a nap**

Legal aspects of sleep and alertness

The legal position of a person whose lack of alertness results in injury depends on the issue of negligence. In principle there is no liability for anything that is done during a period of unconsciousness. Loss caused by a person who is entirely unconscious cannot be recovered from that person, though a claim may be allowed if the person who caused the damage was in some way responsible for allowing himself to become a hazard to others. For example, if a person is aware that he may have an epileptic seizure or some other condition that will cause him to lose consciousness he will be liable for damage that he causes as a result of any loss of consciousness.

Partial loss of consciousness is no defence against an action for damages. As long as the person who caused the damage had some degree of awareness of what was happening, he may be liable. This rule may seem harsh, but it accords with the objective standard of care that the law imposes in which a defendant's individual infirmities are usually not taken into account when assessing liability. To do otherwise would deny compensation to a person who was in no sense responsible for his own loss.

ack of alertness and driving licences

> The fact that narcolepsy and epilepsy are treated similarly as far as driving is concerned perpetuates confusion in the collective consciousness of the lay public, who think that the two conditions must therefore be similar. This is not the case

> In some countries it is the physician's obligation to inform the licensing authorities about potential impairment to drive. A recent court case in Canada in which a doctor was found liable has resulted in the authorities being flooded with reports of "new" cases

In the United Kingdom, a patient who has a condition that will affect his or her ability to drive has a legal obligation to inform the licensing authorities. Prescribed disabilities include not only epilepsy and narcolepsy, but also "sudden attacks of disabling giddiness or fainting." The category embraces loss of consciousness caused by conditions other than epilepsy. Any sleep disorder that causes excessive daytime sleepiness must be notified to the licensing authorities and they will require the patient to stop driving until symptoms are satisfactorily controlled. Licensing will then be subject to regular medical review.

It is an offence for a person to drive in the knowledge that he has a disability about which the authorities should be told. A doctor who is aware that a driver has such a condition should draw attention to the dangers of driving, though the doctor is not under a specific obligation to tell him that he is breaking the law if he continues to drive. There is evidence that many drivers with epilepsy (up to 60%) do not inform the licensing authorities and it may be that a doctor who is aware of a patient in this category may wish to inform the authorities. The breach of confidence involved in such a disclosure may be justified on the grounds of public interest, but an effort should first be made to persuade the patient to inform the authorities and at no time should the information be disclosed except to those who are entitled to know.

Driving and alertness: criminal law

> ## Attorney General's Reference No 2 of 1992
> A lorry driver had driven his heavy goods vehicle some 640 m (700 yards) along the hard shoulder of a motorway. He had not been driving for an excessive length of time, but argued that his alertness had been diminished to the point where he was acting automatically. At the trial, evidence was given by a psychologist to the effect that the driver was "driving without awareness," a condition in which he would be aware of only some aspects of his surroundings. It was stated that a driver in this condition passes into a trance-like state in which the focal point of forward vision comes closer and closer to the windscreen. Peripheral vision continues to function and this allowed the driver to continue to steer.
>
> Though the trial judge allowed a possible defence of automatism to go to the jury, the Court of Appeal ruled that such states do not amount to automatism, and that a driver in such circumstances is criminally responsible for the consequences of his loss of alertness.

Driving long distances along featureless roads may have a pronounced effect on a driver's alertness, and it is quite common for a driver to fall asleep and lose control of the vehicle. The consequences of this may be serious, and criminal prosecution may result if other road users are killed. A recent case in the Court of Appeal in England, *The Attorney General's Reference No 2 of 1992*, illustrates this.

When a driver falls completely asleep at the wheel the courts may convict of a driving offence on the grounds that the driver should have pulled off the road when he started to feel drowsy or if he knew that there were factors that might have caused him to fall asleep. In an important recent case in Australia, the Court of Criminal Appeal of south Australia ruled that though in most cases drivers will have a warning of the onset of sleep, there may be circumstances in which sleep is entirely unpredicted and that in such cases a driver may expect to be acquitted.

Legal aspects of sleep and alertness
Somnambulistic violence and the law

R v Burgess

Somnambulism was treated as insane automatism, which excluded simple acquittal. The accused had fallen asleep while watching a video at a neighbour's house. He awoke to find himself holding his neighbour down on the floor; she had received a serious laceration on the head from blows that he had apparently struck with a bottle and with the video recorder itself. The defence attempted to categorise the assault as an instance of non-insane automatism, but this was unsuccessful.

The Court of Appeal took the view that such behaviour was not caused by an external factor but was, by contrast, the result of the operation of an internal factor. Medical evidence was produced to the effect that somnambulism was associated with an abnormality of brain function and was therefore attributable to a pathological condition. Once this was conceded, the grounds for treating it as insane automatism were established.

Criminal liability normally requires that any person accused of a crime should have committed a voluntary act. Acts which are the result of overwhelming physical force, or which are committed while in a state of automatism (for example, the postictal stage of an epileptic seizure) are considered as involuntary and do not therefore result in criminal conviction. Somnambulistic acts seem to fall into this category because they do not involve conscious control. An act of somnambulistic violence should not then have any criminal consequences because the accused has simply not "acted" in the legal sense. That is the theory; in practice somnambulism involves difficult decisions for the courts, which have as a result responded somewhat ambivalently.

There are two legal forms of automatism. "Insane automatism" exists where the automatic behaviour has resulted from an internal factor (such as arteriosclerosis or epilepsy). "Non-insane automatism" stems from an external factor (such as concussion, when the external factor is the blow that caused the concussion). This distinction is designed to ensure that those who represent a possible social danger are subject to psychiatric supervision or even detention, while those who are not a danger may be unconditionally acquitted. Somnambulistic behaviour is obviously automatic behaviour, but in which category of automatism is it to be placed? This matter has been resolved in English law by the Court of Appeal's decision in *R v Burgess*.

The criminal justice system has, of course, to serve more than one purpose. Not only must it do justice to the person accused of a criminal offence (and therefore avoid convicting those who are not morally responsible for their actions) but it must also serve the legitimate desire of the public for protection. There is a case for psychiatric supervision of those who commit violent acts while asleep. They may not need detention in a psychiatric hospital subject to a restriction order; lesser medical supervision may be quite adequate.

In England this sort of discretion may now be exercised by the court under the *Criminal Procedure (Insanity and Unfitness to Plead) Act 1991*. Insane automatism need no longer inevitably lead to detention in hospital and the court has some less drastic means of recognising the (admittedly remote) risk of future violence. This may take the form of a supervision and treatment order.